EAT LESS, ENJOY MORE

36 Simple Ways to Mindfully Keep Food from Taking Over Your Life

Rachel Zentz

ISBN-13: 978-1727399219
ISBN-10: 1727399218

DEDICATION

I dedicate this book to everyone who has shed tears over their feelings of hopelessness in regard to their eating habits and indulgences. I pray this book brings you the hope you seek.

DOWNLOAD THE AUDIOBOOK FREE!

READ THIS FIRST

Just to say thanks for buying my book,
I would like to give you the
Audiobook version 100% FREE

TO DOWNLOAD GO TO:

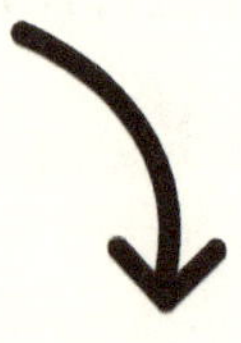

RachelZentz.com/ELEMAudio

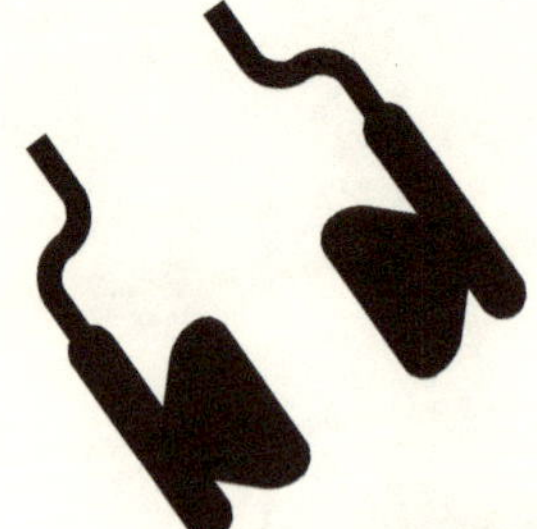

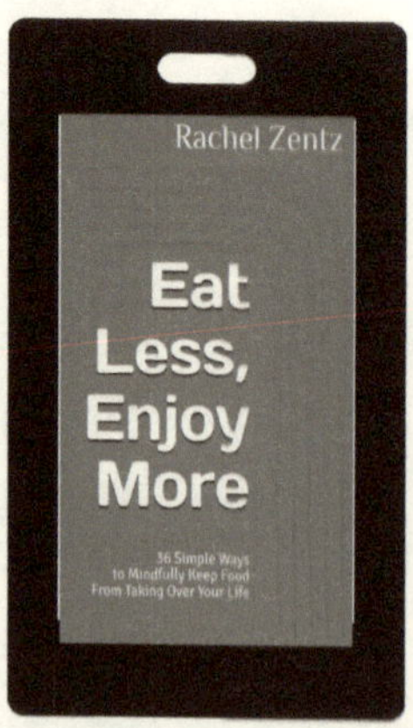

CONTENTS

After Party

Extras

Bonus Chapters

Conclusion

INTRODUCTION

During the movie, I had already decided the first-floor half bath wasn't even an option—people could walk past that door on their way to the kitchen and hear. With the decision made to use the 2nd floor bathroom, I bunched together the 13 Reese's® wrappers and unfolded myself from underneath the fluffy blanket. The blanket protected me from the chill in the house, but it did nothing for my shame and guilt.

My teenage mind and focus began to cloud, as it did every time I succumbed to a temptation or ate too much. Keeping up appearances, I walked up the carpeted steps, even though my foggy mind told me to run so I could put this all behind me as fast as possible.

I ascended the final step, walked straight into the bathroom, closed and locked the door behind me. I grabbed my aunt's toothbrush from the holder on the sink, turned it upside down in my right hand, raised the toilet seat lid, knelt in front of it, and held my hair back with my left hand while I puked out the sweet taste of shame and guilt.

FACING THE CHANGE

As a high schooler, I was experimenting with ways to deal with my overeating habit. I didn't know what I was feeling, why I was feeling it, or what to do about it. I had heard vomiting was something some people were doing, so I thought I'd give it a try. Fortunately, I did not like this experience and only tried it a handful of times.

While your experience and reaction to overeating the wrong foods may be different than my high school experience, there may still be something you feel you need to change or do differently in regard to eating habits you've grown into over the years.

Maybe it's eating right before you sleep. Maybe it's eating too quickly. Maybe it's "checking out" while you're eating dessert, so you don't have to face it. Maybe it's loading up your plate buffet-style. Maybe it's skipping meals. Maybe it's feeling like every single time you give into a temptation, you feel like you failed (Yes, mindset is a habit that can be changed.). Maybe it's skipping breakfast. Maybe it's just not being willing to totally give up sweets but knowing something has to change about them. Maybe you take an "eat now, don't-think-about-it later" approach rather than a more controlled "plan now, then eat."

It's extremely hard to admit—and even more difficult to face—the feeling of not being able to control a bad eating habit. Add on the knowledge of *needing* to change it and not knowing where to start—or even if you want to—and *avoiding* the whole subject becomes so much easier than trying to face it and fix it.

FREE FROM FEARING FOOD

The perfect way to start gaining momentum, confidence, and control is to start small with easy strategies that don't totally disrupt your life. Feeling on top of your eating game puts the defeating self-talk and shaming thoughts to rest, allowing you to concentrate more fully on other, more important, aspects of life.

I am going to walk you through all of the strategies, tips, and tricks that are ultra-effective at getting you to eat *less* while still eating what you *love* while enjoying it even *more* without "dieting." Taking back control has never been so sweet—literally.

My mission is simple: to help people be the best, happiest, most energetic and positive version of themselves. We start with eating habits…

SETTING THE STAGE

1

BULKING

The best preparation for tomorrow is doing your best today.
—H. JACKSON BROWN, JR

The goal is to cut back on the bad foods yet still be able to enjoy them. Some may need to be cut out completely, sure. But we don't want to feel restricted. Thus, learning moderation is key as we are adopting and learning a new way of eating.

We are hard workers, and we all like to be sure we are getting the best and most use out of our dollar. Buying things in bulk is usually more inexpensive, thrifty, cheap, economical—whatever word you like to use—for the long term. The per-unit cost within the bulk package is typically less than if you purchased that same unit individually or in a smaller package.

RULE

Make it a rule to purchase veggies, lean meats and fish, and anything else healthy in bulk. Look for the largest container or bag they sell. Make sure to compare the price per ounce on the price tag on the shelf to be sure it truly is the best value (every once in while you will find an item that is not).

You can freeze the veggies if you do not use them before they go bad, or you can get bulk bags of already frozen veggies, already cut and washed, and ready for your steamer or casserole. Lean meats come in bulk packages that are easily divided. Use a freezer Ziploc® baggie, which are available in a large variety of sizes, to divide your meats into single-use meals, such as four chicken breasts for a family of two or four (leftover chicken is amazing).

WHEN TO NOT BUY IN BULK

Treats and other unhealthy items are the items to *not* buy in bulk, even though they are 99.9% of the time less expensive to buy in bulk.

That's ridiculous, why would I want to do that?

In summary, it helps to *un*-justify cost. I was at the store about a month ago, and one of the items my husband requested was Oreos. They had a special: 2 packages for Oreos for $5 while a single package was $2.99. I chose the single.

Allow me to explain with my three rationales. Let's use the oh-so-chocolatey-goodness of Oreos as the example (by the way, side note, did you know there are 47 different varieties of Oreos?):

> 1— Imagine a family-sized package of Oreos and a regular size package. A regular package of Oreos currently has 3 rows of 12 cookies. A family-size package of Oreos has 3 rows of 16 cookies. You get the family-size package. It's quite easy to play mind games with yourself, saying you only ate one row of cookies, but if the package is larger with

longer rows, that little mind game is completely defeating you; you just ate 33% more Oreos as you would have if you had gotten the smaller package, even though you can still say you only ate one row. Add in the confounding factor of the thicker (and thus taking up more room in the package) Double Stuf, and you have a real brain twister on your hands.

(Side note: As scrumptious as Oreos are, I do *not* condone eating an entire row of Oreos. This was simply an example given to prove a point.)

2— By purchasing the treats in sizes that are more expensive per treat, it associates the purchasing of said treat with a *negative* cost analysis ($.20 per Oreo in a package of 6 cookies), rather than the *positive* affirmation that you just got a screaming deal ($.05 per cookie in a bulk box of 132 Oreos). Make the treat more *expensive.* In this way, it truly is a *treat,* in part because by purchasing the smaller container, it is more expensive.

3— This kind of purchasing makes the treat more of a delicacy. If you only have a 6-pack of Oreos, you likely will only have 2 or 3 to be able to save the rest for another day. If you have a 132-count bulk box, eating 10 in one sitting barely makes a dent in the container. Mind games, my friend, mind games.

It's like if you only have $6 in your checking account until payday in 2 days, that $4 snack you are about to purchase will make a huge dent in your $6 balance and seem unnecessary, and you most likely will opt for a $1 snack instead... or... eat half of that snack and save the rest for tomorrow. However, if you have $132 in your checking, that $4 snack will hardly make a dent, and you likely will not even think twice about handing your debit card over. It is the same $4 snack, but your perspective changes dramatically when the circumstances are altered.

Just like the Oreo. It is the same three Oreos, but your perspective changes dramatically when the total number of Oreos you have (i.e. the circumstances) are altered or changed.

Make that treat a rare, limited commodity. It will also prompt you to relish and savor it because you know it is limited.

This is does not mean you buy 10 6-count packages of Oreos. No sir, you buy one at a time, thereby forcing the three rationales above while still allowing you your treat.

RECAP

Buy healthy items in bulk. Buy treats in small, *un*-economical packages, one at a time.

2

TEMPTING

Don't wait. The time will never be just right.
—NAPOLEON HILL

Heck no, you don't want to be a lifetime yo-yo dieter and go on 3-month bouts of deprivation of everything but water and veggies. What kind of fun is that? The best thing to do is live a life of healthy eating that serves you and your body for years and years. However, you also don't want to keep purchasing *all* the junk and keep eating like before.

It is much easier to binge-eat *all* the crappy foods if they are readily accessible to you, in your house, staring you in the face, with no healthy options even available to you. If there is an item that calls to you in your kitchen that when you want a snack, you think of this quick, satisfying food, *and* the tips, tricks, and tactics thus far haven't helped with this particular food, it may be time for a more drastic change. Here are some options:

1. Throw it away. This is my least favorite option, but you have to do what you have to do.

2. Donate it. If it is unopened, this is an option. Donate to a shelter or other cause, or even just to a friend or neighbor. At least then it's not getting wasted.

3. Freeze it. Set rules for yourself that allow you to have the treat you decide on, but create a rule for how much. Never eat tempting, unhealthy foods from a bulk bag or box of seemingly endless supply of said treat. This makes it way too difficult to gauge how much you have eaten, which inevitably leads to overeating and guilt. Freezing it may be an odd option—if it's still in your house, you could still eat it, right? Well, not usually if it's frozen. Always freeze it in single-serving sizes, and when you do allow yourself that treat, pull only one portion out to thaw at a time. By the time you take it out of the freezer, let it thaw, and have your glass of water like we have already discussed, your cravings may be gone or significantly reduced. Or another option is to only thaw it when company is over. That way you are not wasting it or your money, but you are saving it for another time and another use and for other people.

RECAP

You don't need discipline if you remove temptation.

3

90–10

Only I can change my life. No one can do it for me.
—CAROL BURNETT

So I know I need to do something *better, and Rachel, you said I could have treats and desserts and alcohol and cheeseburgers, but how do I know or monitor how much?* I'll attack the "how do I know how much" now and the "how do I monitor" in a later chapter.

HOW MUCH

Everyone responds to various food differently and fluctuates weight differently; one approach or lifestyle will not necessarily affect two people in the same way. For this reason, experimenting—and patience—will be necessary.

A safe rule of thumb that I live by is to take the approach of a 90/10 way of eating. A healthy balance is key, so the "90—10" refers to 90% of the time you are eating healthy foods that fuel your body in the right portions. Society's acceptance of "healthy" isn't quite what I mean here. Transitioning from regular soda to "diet" soda is absolutely *not* healthy and not part of the 90%. "Healthy food" references food that will *give* you energy rather than bog you down. Healthy food that is simply made and minimally processed with simple, real ingredients.

Since balance—not restriction—is the focus, 10% of the time you are allowing yourself the glaringly unhealthy alternatives while keeping appropriate portions, of course, and remembering every other tip contained within this book. Remember, we are figuring out a healthy relationship with food and eating. We are figuring out a way of eating that you can keep for the rest of your life.

GLARINGLY UNHEALTHY

I use the term "glaringly" because I am talking about the obvious bad foods—the cakes, sodas ("diet" included), cookies, deep-fried foods, thick sauces and creams, fatty red meats, etc. For instance, accessorizing a salad with cheese is not ideal, but the 10% I am talking about in *this* instance does *not* apply to accessories such as those. Completely *drenching* a salad with processed, lard-based, creamy, calorie-laden dressing on top of a salad *is*.

EATING FOR FUEL

Food is meant to fuel and energize your mind and body for everything it does for you. You know the feeling you have when you drink an extra cup of coffee your body does not usually get? I am talking about the feeling of being alert, being able to quickly and clearly shift your thinking and speaking, to take in everything going on around you, of feeling light and energized? Do you get a sense of accomplishment... a proud feeling... a done feeling... when you are able to efficiently get the things you need to take care of done for the day and do it well? When you are able to prioritize and plan for the next day and week so clearly that everything makes sense?

Crappy, overly processed foods take that all away from us. Our bodies have to go into overdrive to digest and allocate the man-made ingredients we feed it, taking the resources from other places, like our brains and muscles. Enjoying those donuts for those 5 minutes is a large price to pay for hours of zapped energy.

I personally hate having a foggy mind and a heavy, tired body. You have to ask yourself, is it worth the 5 minutes of sugary yumminess to feel like that for hours? Choose your 10% wisely, and pay attention to how these foods make you feel and perform an hour later. The more you pay attention, the more you may find it not even being worth it to eat the crap as often.

RECAP

Adopt a 90—10 mentality that is nonrestrictive and yet still benefiting your body; 90% of what you consume is healthy to your body, and 10% can be fun and silly treats, bad carbs, and drinks.

4

CLOTHING

If you fell down yesterday, stand up today.
—H.G. WELLS

While coaching people through their nutrition and fitness journey, I encounter many people who have a goal of firming up their mid-section, especially as the Spring and Summer months approach. For varying reasons, there seems to be a heightened sensitivity in regard to the belly region, especially in the warmer months when fewer layers are needed and swimsuits are common.

Fewer layers and tighter clothing seems to make most people more aware of their bodies. If large, comfy sweatshirts and sweaters are worn most days, awareness of and thoughts about the tummy region are minimized.

Overeating makes your stomach bulge. It doesn't matter your size, weight, or gender. It happens to everyone. The reduced awareness is also reflected in the amount of food—and subsequent stomach bulging—that is consumed.

I have noticed people are much more aware of how much food they eat if the clothes are more form-fitting, and conversely it's much easier to overeat in comfy, poufy clothes.

I'm not saying this tactic will work for everyone, but I *am* saying give it a try. Next time you go out for dinner, meet a coworker for lunch, or eat a sit-down meal solo, wear a tighter, form-fitting shirt and/or pants and notice if it makes you more aware of how much you are eating.

RECAP

Try wearing smaller-size or more form-fitting clothes.

5

PRE-SNACKING

What you plant now, you will harvest later.
—OG MANDINO

If you could do one super simple thing to help you lose weight and feel more energetic *aaaand* it's free, would you do it? Of course! Before you put *anything* in your mouth, whether it be a meal, a handful of mints, or a soda, make a rule for yourself that you *must* drink a full 8 ounces of water first.

Drinking a full 8 ounces of water before your meal or snack serves many, many purposes, four of which I want to highlight. Knowing the *why* will help to motivate you to actually put the effort forth to carry it out.

HYDRATION

1— Duh. It keeps you hydrated. One of your goals is—or should be—to stay hydrated. How much water, you may ask. What kinds of liquids, you may ask. Take your current body weight and divide by half. This is the number of ounces at the *minimum* you must be drinking for a sedentary lifestyle. You guessed it; that number only goes up the more active you are and the warmer the conditions in which you spend your day. If you make it a rule to drink at least a full glass of water before every meal and snack, you will be doing very well in hitting your minimum daily water requirement.

REDUCE CRAVINGS

2— It reduces cravings. Many people live their lives mildly dehydrated without even knowing it. Seriously, *most* people. Probably even you. Your mouth may not feel dry, and your body may feel "normal" to you because that *is* your normal. One of the byproducts of dehydration are misaligned cravings. By drinking a full glass of water before every meal and snack, some of these cravings are thwarted.

FULLNESS

3— It starts the fullness effect. Have you ever overeaten a delicious meal, and you seriously feel like you can't take another bite? I am guessing drinking a full glass of water in that instance is close to impossible as well, and definitely not something you even want to consider. That is because water adds to your fullness effect. If you drink this *before* you eat, you will most likely eat less. Smart, right?!

DELAY CRAVINGS

4— It will delay the craving. If you keep this "rule" a staple during your day, the craving you are having or mindless eating to which you are about to succumb will be delayed by the time it takes to gulp the 8 ounces. This serves two purposes: 1— The extra 8 ounces of water may help to curb your craving. 2— It gives you time to reflect on that food and reevaluate if it is what you truly want and need, or if it is something to ease the boredom, ease the stress, ease the loneliness, or any other non-hunger related reason for which you were going to indulge yourself.

21

RECAP

Drink water. Think of it as your pre-appetizer. Another simple one. Wow.

6

GRUMBLING

I got no time for the jibba-jabba.
—MR. T

It's a metabolism thing. It's a mind thing. It's an energy thing. It's a moderation thing. It's a planning thing. It's a preparedness thing.

I was a school psychologist for a school district, and a significant component of my workday was meetings, many of which I led. How could I think about my hunger when I was leading a 2-hour meeting with school administration, teachers, and parents?

By anticipating the length of the meeting ahead of time and assessing my level of hunger the hour before the meeting, yes, I was busy prepping, but I could have had an easy-to-snack-on snack, like nuts, on my desk as I was doing my thing.

STARVATION MODE

The longer you keep your body hungry, the more it will adapt to being in a "starvation mode." Your body is very adaptable with its main goal of keeping you alive. If it is not getting nutrition (a.k.a. fuel) often enough to keep it going and running smoothly, it starts to recognize this and begins to store fat in your body in anticipation for future periods of no food. Survival is the name of the game.

One of the first things people, especially young people, go to when they feel they need to "lose weight," is cutting out meals and snacks all together. Except in extreme cases of clinically-severe disordered eating, in all honesty, this will get you results quickly, but it also will not last. It just can't. Your body will soon adapt and start protecting itself against these periods of no food by storing what it needs to keep all of the processes going in your body. Your body does so much for you that you are not even aware of, and it needs a consistent stream of good-for-you food—energy and nutrients—to be able to sustain those processes optimally.

REACTIVE MODE

Listen to your body. Don't ignore those hunger pains. Feed your body when it needs food. If it is hungry—not *cravings* hungry—but legitimately hunger-pains-hungry, feed it the fuel it needs. There is a lot going on inside your body to make all of your organs, systems, and even cells work how they should. And they need to two things to do that... two very simple things: Fuel and water. That's all they need to keep you operating at your best and to keep you feeling your best.

It seems like the "feeling" part gets pushed behind the "looking" part. But it absolutely sucks and is greatly frustrating to feel drained, fuzzy, or unfocused. Give your body the absolute best, so you don't feel like crap. When you feel like crap, everything around you tends to go to crap. You lose perspective on important things which makes you short, irritable, unmotivated, and low on energy. You subsequently do less, plan less, get the important things accomplished less, snap on people you love more, let your goals go down the toilet because you can't concentrate on them, go into reactive mode rather than proactive mode, and nothing of meaning or substance gets done. *And* you eat more, usually of the foods that are more convenient, quick, and unhealthy. All because your body could not function because it was initially fed crap... or not fed at all.

Once you get into a routine of eating consistently throughout the day, your body will adjust and think, oh I am getting fed exactly when I need the fuel, and it will then start burning that fuel and using that it much quicker (instead of storing it for when you starve your body) for the processes it needs it for.

BINGE MODE

You may be thinking, *Rachel, this is a book about eating less, and you are telling me to eat more often... what's up with that?*

Skipping meals greatly enhances the likelihood that you will eat much more during the next meal you do not skip. Think back to last time you were "starving." Didn't just about *everything* sound yummy and appetizing to you? This is one of the reasons there is sound advice out there warning us to not grocery shop while we are hungry.

When you feel you are "starving" because of skipped meals or going many hours without eating, when we do get food, we take much larger bites, chew less, pay attention less, eat faster, and eat *more* than we would otherwise. Then your body stores more of it because it's used to you going long periods of time without giving it what it needs (food).

RECAP

If you are truly hungry, give your body healthy food. Don't skip meals or snacks. Give it crap, you will feel like crap, your body will not be fed what it needs to thrive, you will not function at your best, you will go into reactive mode (as opposed to proactive), and you will eat more, most likely of the bad stuff you wish you hadn't.

7

MORNING

Nothing is impossible. The word itself says, "I'm possible!"
—AUDREY HEPBURN

We have heard that breakfast is the most important meal of the day. Eating within an hour of waking gets you out of the slumber-imposed fast your body just endured. I am not recommending *what* to eat—if you read the introduction to this book, you know that is not what this book is about—I *am* recommending, however, that you *do* eat, however small or large, carbs or proteins, fruits or veggies, there are many opinions out there about what is best, and I am not here to pretend I am an expert in the *what*... but I am here to tell you to just eat *something* to get your body going. It will kick your metabolism in the pants, and once your body is in the habit of expecting and relying on food within an hour of you waking up, it will know it can safely use it for fuel, rather than having to store it in fear you will starve your body by going hours upon hours of not eating.

The only recommendation I am giving about the *what* is to know what is best for your body. You want sustained energy, right? The best carbohydrate to consume in the morning is one that is a long-term energy source, rather than one that will drop off quickly and leave you feeling like you were hit by a freight train an hour later. Mid-morning slump... no thank you. I'm guessing you want a type of food that will keep you feeling full until you at least get to your first mid-morning meeting and not have you reaching for that donut as you first walk into the office.

Not only that, but to skip breakfast is to skip a meal... is to go an even longer time without food... is to get more and more hungry... is to feel famished... is to then binge and eat fast and whatever is first available that even remotely resembles food.

The longer you go without eating, the more likely you are to overeat.

RECAP

Plan to eat breakfast. However big or small. Do your research to know what is best. That's it. Carry on.

8

TASTING

You'll never change your life until you change something you do daily. The secret of your success is found in your daily routine.
—JOHN C MAXWELL

I am saying this to you with the utmost respect because I know you want to change. You want to learn. You want to experiment. But you may not be open to certain types of foods, like salad, for instance, because of the *taste*. Whole grain bread may not be an option because of the *taste*. You don't buy the superfood smoothies because you're afraid they won't *taste* good.

TASTE CAN BE AN ENEMY

Friend, "*taste*" is probably what got you in trouble in the first place. Of course, the cakes and candies and fries and cheese curds are more tasty. The depth of their flavor far outweighs that of salad or whole grain bread.

But also know that *taste* is learned. Taste preferences are acquired, wholly dependent on what we—and our taste buds—are used to.

That is the *good* news… we can *change* it. You have to change it if *you* want to change. You cannot 100% of the time go by taste anymore. I can't tell you how many people have told me they don't want to try another health shake because they have tried others and don't like the "*taste*." It is just another way to not have to try anymore and say, *I guess this healthy thing just isn't for me. I'm just made this way. I will always be this way.*

I call bullshit. That is an excuse. You have control over your mind.

The less you eat the greasy, oily, sugary, creamy, salty, rich foods, the *less* you will come to expect them, and the *less* you will be feeling like something is missing when they are not present in the foods you are eating. For instance, if you go through the 3-Day Refresh™ which gives you a 3-day prescriptive and timed eating regimen with a menu of foods you choose based on preference, you will finish that not only with some pounds lost, but also with a very different perspective of food and a shift and recalibration, if you will, of your taste buds. You *can* change what you are used to tasting and therefore what you like and don't like.

It is all what you are *used* to, and until you understand both that… and that it *can* be altered to not even want or crave the bad stuff anymore… aaaaand be open to trying to 'recalibrate,' you will always be stuck in the same place. You *can* change. You *can* learn to like foods you presently have a closed mind about. You have to open your mind to new possibilities, or everything will stay the same.

RECAP

Your taste preferences and being stubborn about what you do and do not 'like' can be a sneaky, relentless, weight-adding factor… but is also one you control and change.

9

CHANGING

If you are brave enough to say, "Goodbye,"
life will reward you with a new, "Hello."
—PAULO COELHO

Imagine rearranging the furniture or wall décor in a room in your house. You walk in that room for the first time after it has been changed, and it feels like a whole other room. You take notice of things you didn't before and hadn't in a long time.

As room accessories have become "normal" and expected over the months and years, you most likely tended to glaze right past certain aspects and features of the furniture, decorations, and/or room that have had for years… because they stayed the same. Your notice of, focus on, and appreciation for those aspects of the room are diminished now because they are an expected part of your house and room arrangement. But hang a new shelf on a previously bare wall and move a picture frame from a bookcase to that new shelf on the wall, and all of a sudden, it's like a whole new addition to the room, even though that frame is years old. You notice it every time you walk into the room, at least for the first few days. Your focus shifts from everything swirling around inside your mind to that shelf and picture frame because it's unexpected and not the norm.

You immerse yourself in the presence and feel of the room because of the newness.

MEALS

You may be able to apply this same logic to changes to your eating habits as well. When disrupted and changed, a new facet of your previously "normal" eating pattern can open up a whole new dimension of focusing on and enjoying your food and will help to diminish the mindless eating or eating out of habit rather than necessity or hunger. When your expected routine is shifted or disrupted by implementing some sort of change, your habits and what you are used to doing without really thinking is forced to change and snap into awareness.

By this I do not mean eat *more;* I mean *savor,* so you are more satiated and satisfied sooner into your meal and thereby eat less but still enjoy it more. Some changes I am referring to are the location within your house or workplace that you typically consume your meals, the time of day and/or frequency of your meals, the types of utensils you use, and/or the types of food or the way they are prepared or cooked.

Whether you like change or not, in the world of your eating habits, changing something up and disrupting your routine can be a welcome and useful disruption to your normal routine.

RECAP

Implement a change to your eating pattern, such as time, frequency, type, preparation, location, and/or method.

10

BRUSHING

Dentists have recommended brushing your teeth at least two times a day—when you wake and before bed—as a part of a healthy oral hygiene regimen. Optimally, brush your teeth after every meal, especially if you have braces.

What I am suggesting, though, is different.

BEFORE MEALS

What I am suggesting is to brush your teeth *before* your meal. This will "reset" your mouth and palate. You will be able to more fully taste your food and not have cravings from tastes that were already in your mouth.

Haven't you ever had something salty and then craved a sweet treat? Or vice versa—had something sweet and craved a salty snack an hour later? Particles of food stay in your mouth and on your tongue and gums long after you have eaten, coating your mouth in gross bacteria and ickiness. Get rid of all that and reset your palate by brushing your teeth before eating.

DURING CRAVINGS

When you are hit with a 'sweet tooth' or you get that routine sweet craving after dinner, try brushing your teeth *before* you succumb to the craving. Sweet and sour foods will become altered in flavor and less appeasing for about 30 minutes after you brush your teeth. You can thank the foaming agent in your toothpaste for that. It will help rid you of your sweet craving.

AFTER THE LAST MEAL

To help curb the late-night snacking, don't wait until right before bed to brush. Be sure to brush those pearly whites immediately after the last meal of the day. This genius little trick will not only signal to your brain that eating and drinking anything but water is done for the day, but it will alter the taste of any sweet snacks you indulge in, negatively reinforcing that habit in the future.

RECAP

Brush your teeth before you eat, when cravings strike, and immediately after the last meal of the day. You will most likely eat less, enjoy the food you do eat more, and be signaled sooner in the evening that eating is done for the day.

11

PLATING

Start where you are. Use what you have. Do what you can.
—ARTHUR ASHE

Maybe your random dishware you hardly ever use is *just* what the doctor ordered. Do you have a couple random dishes left over from your last set in the back of your cabinet? Or maybe two different sized plates in your current set? Maybe a salad plate and a dinner-sized plate? Or do you have saucers with cute little tea cups your Aunt Minnie gave you that you never use? How about the full set of silverware you got for your wedding with the tiny forks and tiny spoons that never gets brought out?

MIND GAMES

Satiety, or the perceived feeling of fullness, is as much a mental game as it is a physical one. Try switching to these tinier versions of the dishes and utensils for your meals.

The same amount of food—the same sized portions—look larger and taller on a small plate... and smaller and shorter on a big plate.

This goes for your bowls, glasses, forks, and spoons as well. Beverages seem larger when in thinner, smaller cups as opposed to the gigantic plastic cups you used in college or at picnics. For some of you, you focus on the mound of food. Your mind automatically assumes that, when the same amount of food is placed on a large plate, you are eating less because it *looks* smaller compared to the large plate. Conversely, when that same amount of food is placed on a small plate, you assume you are eating more because it looks larger compared to the small plate.

This logic won't be as effective for some of you, however, because you focus on the plate size. Just *knowing* the size of the plate will play into your mental game. You people will automatically think you are eating less *just* because it is on a smaller plate, even if it does include a larger portion than what would be on your larger plate.

What kind of person are *you*? Give it a try. You don't have to buy more plates... at least not yet. Consider using a saucer or a salad plate that you already have in place of your usual dinner plate. Drink beverages other than water out of a smaller coffee cup instead of your large drinking glasses.

If you absolutely do not have anything smaller than what you already use, go to a department store and just purchase one smaller sized plate, bowl, and cup in a color or pattern that you would buy an entire set of if you could. Or maybe buy a plastic one to experiment with and then donate it to your camping box once your little experiment is over. If you want to try it out with a less expensive option, hit up your local thrift shop or dollar store; they have sturdy, plastic dishes and utensils in sets of four. Whatever you decide, just give it a try for a week, and see what happens.

RECAP

Try the smaller dishes and utensils for a week. If they are working for you in terms of encouraging you to eat less, it's time to switch over full time. If you don't have a full set of the small stuff, it's time to invest.

12

USING TOOLS

> *Knowing is not enough; we must apply.*
> *Willing is not enough; we must do.*
> —BRUCE LEE

We gobble. We gulp. And then we go. We know it's bad. We do it anyway.

We have talked about many ways around this with a primary theme of bringing your focus back to what you are doing: *eating*.

Another idea is to try using a different tool—even if just for a week—to force you to slow down and appreciate your food. Newness is an aspect that can force you to take notice. Let's use it to our advantage in our quest to be more mindful of what and how we are eating, eat less, and enjoy it more.

IDEAS

Have you ever used chopsticks? How about trying to eat with your non-dominant hand?

If you are not used to chopsticks and are not ambidextrous, this could be quite funny, entertaining, and challenging at the same time. You definitely would have to focus in on your food and the eating process to successfully eat using these tactics.

The goal is appreciating what you are eating so you don't eat as much and yet can still gain satisfaction and enjoyment.

Use a spoon in place of a fork. Use a fork in place of a spoon. Anything to slow yourself down and reintroduce the element of surprise and newness to your food. Try using a knife as your fork. Use a different water container. Use a smaller glass for your beverage, unless it is water.

RECAP

Try a different tool or utensil to eat. Yes, it may be ridiculous, but it will accomplish the purpose of forcing you to focus on, slow down with, and appreciate what you are consuming with the ultimate goal being that you will have more control

13

PORTIONING

*I can't change the direction of the wind, but I can adjust my sails
to always reach my destination.*
—JIMMY DEAN

Have you ever eaten ice cream right out of the container? Or dunked your veggie in the container of hummus? Or got the best deal on the bulk bag of trail mix but then ate half the bag in one day? Or how about the pan of brownies that are almost gone? Or grabbed the whole container of cottage cheese to eat out of instead of dirtying another bowl? Or how about grabbed the whole bag of chips to munch out of?

Sure thing! I know I do it. After you think you may be done, you convince yourself, just a little bit more. Or tell yourself, *Well, it's almost gone now, might as well finish it off.*

RULE

Tell yourself as of right now, no more eating out of any containers or bulk bags that are *more* than one serving. Take the time to get a clean plate or bowl to ration that food item *before* you dig in.

Reference the nutritional table on the container first to find out exactly how much of that food item is one serving. For instance, ice cream is usually measured by cups, hummus by tablespoons, chips by number of chips, and so on.

BENEFITS

The single-sized portion is in front of you. The container is put away. You are much more able and willing to pace yourself and make doubly sure you enjoy it because it's not a seemingly bottomless container.

You are taking control by deciding how much you are going to eat *before* you start digging in to the yumminess, and you know *exactly* how much you did eat once you're finished. If you keep a food journal, this will make it much easier, and it will eliminate the gorging, which leads to the mindless overeating, which leads to the guilt, which leads to self-shaming.

RECAP

Portion one serving size of your food as indicated on the nutrition label, and put the remaining away *before* you begin to eat your portion.

14

SPACING

They always say time changes things,
but you actually have to change them yourself.
—ANDY WARHOL

Sometimes the little quirks of childhood come back to benefit us as adults.

As adults, we tend to pile our plates with the foods we enjoy, and the pile is able to be larger the more we allow the different food items rest on each other. Additionally, when it's the same plate used year after year, you become accustomed to filling it higher and higher, piling on and overlapping the food.

HERE'S THE DEAL

Remember when you were a kid, and you had that friend that hated it if any of her food touched any other type of food on her plate? Maybe you didn't know someone like that, but I did. I always thought it was immensely silly, but now as an adult who wants to cut back on her gorging, it makes perfect sense.

Want to start becoming accustomed to eating less without starving or feeling deprived? Make a rule...

When eating at home and filling your plate with the various parts of your dinner or meal like you've always done, but now make it a rule to not let any type of food touch the other.

This rule or guideline you develop and implement should include the stipulation of being able to see the bottom of your plate around each type of food you are eating. For instance, say you are having a piece of roast, mashed potatoes, and broccoli for your dinner. Each of those should be placed on the plate in separate little mounds with room in between each mound of food.

You are still eating off of the same plate you have been for years, but because the food is not all clumped together in a heap, you are eating less than what you would otherwise have eaten.

THE POINT

The point of this is *not* to develop some sort of phobia or weird obsession thing. The point *is* to help you implement an easy method of keeping your portions under control. Please note, this is definitely *not* the best way to keep your portions at an appropriate size. However, it *is* a start that you can begin to implement immediately without further instruction, learning, or dieting.

In adhering to this 'rule,' you will be more inclined to take forkfuls of each type of food separately, thus allowing you to appreciate each type of food you are eating separate from the others and not mangling them all together in your mouth.

Trail mix is an excellent example. All trail mixes are a little different, but commonly included in the mixes are a variety of nuts and seeds like almonds, peanuts, cashews, and sunflower seeds. There is usually also a variety of sweet ingredients as well, such as raisins, dried fruits, and chocolate candies. When my husband eats trail mix, he pours a half dollar-sized amount into his hand and dumps that small handful into his mouth, mixing the various nuts, seeds, raisins, and dried fruit in his mouth. I wonder how he is able to taste and appreciate all the wonderfulness that makes the trail mix.

Why? You *deserve* to get the full experience and have the satisfaction and enjoyment from your food. This is one way to allow you that pleasure. This is especially useful at holiday mealtimes when overeating is a super common occurrence with the pre-meal snacking and the plethora of choices for the main meal. Feel free to choose all of them, but keep this "rule" in mind as you take spoonfuls of each dish. This will keep your plateful limited but still be considered a plateful, letting you eat less and enjoy more.

...Just don't go back for seconds.

RECAP

Implement a 'rule' for yourself that you must see the plate around all edges of each individual food item you place on your plate without using a larger plate.

15

SITTING

Either you run the day, or the day runs you.
—JIM ROHN

A rule of thumb to implement: I will only eat while I am sitting.

IT'S A MIND GAME

The norm is to sit in a comfortable chair at a table of some sort when eating. When you eat while standing, it automatically tricks your brain into thinking you are in a hurry, even if you truly are not. Consequently, you assume you have less time to eat, no matter how much time you actually do have. You tend to take larger bites, spend less time chewing, and grab whatever is available to eat easily, often less favorable choices.

Eating *more* and enjoying it *less* is usually the outcome. Afterward, you know you aren't exactly *hungry*, per se, but you still *want* food because you didn't get the usual satisfaction from the food you did eat.

SUPER BUSY

Your brain is *immensely* powerful and can trick your body into all sorts of things. It is not nearly as satisfied by the whole standing-while-eating process as when you are sitting and taking your time, and it adds extra stress on our already strained bodies and minds. By not paying attention to the eating process—if you chow down in a hurry—it will almost feel as if you haven't actually eaten because you didn't receive the enjoyment out of the experience to which you are accustomed.

I am definitely guilty of this as well, for varying reasons, depending on the situation and the type of food. So, I am fully aware how hectic life can be with the kids and the work and the chores and the errands and the commitments... but this is *you* we are talking about.

I know it seems selfish and counterproductive to take care of you and to allow yourself time for you, but if you do that, it will allow you to be much more effective and present at taking care of all the rest of the stuff. Not to lump your children into "stuff" or anything, but all of the other responsibilities will seem that much easier to manage and will go more smoothly when you don't feel like *you* are shorted. You will be more grounded, more focused, and feel more in control if you do *you* first.

MINDLESS EATING

Standing while eating unconsciously relays to your brain, let's get this over with as soon as possible so I can move on to the next thing. Enter mindless eating, taking huge bites, swallowing before it should be swallowed, and not fully appreciating the food other than the fact it is filling the void that was in your stomach. Your mind deserves the break to eat the food and enjoy it.

YOU'RE THE COOK

Eating while you are standing often happens when you are preparing and cooking a meal. It's innocent enough, right? You are the one preparing and cooking the meal, so you should get the first taste, or you should make sure it's seasoned properly. Before you know it, you end up consuming a portion of your meal before you actually sit down to eat it. You subsequently feel as if you are doing well by actually eating less at the sit-down meal when in reality, you consumed *more* overall than your normal amount. If you are going to sample the meal or you need a little snack to tide you over until the meal is done, put a tiny taste on a plate, grab a utensil, sit down, and *taste* it.

GUILTY TREATS

Enter a situation that leaves you feeling guilty. There's a treat you love. You see it. You can almost taste it as your mouth begins to water. Just a little taste.

You grab the tray, put it on the kitchen counter, take the top off, grab a fork, lean your hip against countertop, and dip the fork into the cake you actually got for your husband for his birthday two days ago. Just a bite or two to have a taste, right?

Does it *really* ever end up only being one or two bites?

I *know* because I have *done* this... as recently as two days ago... with cake... that I got for my husband.

Psshh, it doesn't really count since I'm just having a few bites... that turned into *eight* very large bites eaten very quickly so I hardly noticed I'm eating them. It makes me feel better... less guilty. It's much better than grabbing a plate and cutting a whole piece... right? Because then it counts. And I know I really would feel guilty about a whole piece of cake. This I don't have to. ...or do I?

See... Our mind is tricky, and the quicker you can train yourself to start catching those sneaky little thoughts, habits, and excuses, and *actually* think about your thoughts that lead to your behaviors, the quicker you will gain control over your food for life.

RECAP

When you eat anything, sit down.

If you want to live a happy life, tie it to a goal,
not people or things.
—Albert Einstein

MAIN EVENT

Whatever you are, be a good one.
—Abraham Lincoln

16

BITING

There is nothing impossible to him who will try.
—ALEXANDER THE GREAT

You know the saying, less is more? I don't know where it comes from or what it refers to, except I know I have heard it used in terms of gift-giving. In terms of food, however, that's not the case. Less is just less. More is just more. And if you know you struggle with overeating, binging, and/or eating too quickly, less is also better.

Digestion begins in the mouth with the salivary glands. Large bites that are not chewed and broken down enough in the mouth will be more difficult for your stomach to break down, which can lead to indigestion, heartburn, and other intestinal and stomach problems.

EXCITEMENT

People are hungry. People get excited. People love food. I am "people" too, and I definitely get it. Especially with pizza and doughnuts and chimichangas and wine to just name a few. Because of that excitement, people have developed ways of satisfying that hunger quickly in all their excitement and love for food.

For instance, in order to take a larger bite, people draw their lips back to expose more of their teeth—almost like a wolf baring its teeth on its prey—and allow their jaw to open wider. This is so they can take a larger, deeper bite.

Awareness is the first step to changing a habit. Since this would be a habit most people have never even thought of, just you reading this is a good first step to controlling this facet of your eating habits.

Do some reflection while eating. Be intentional and cognizant of how your mouth is formed when you take a bite, either off a utensil or as you bite into what you are eating. When you bare your teeth, it is to allow a larger amount of food to go into your mouth.

Large bites = eat faster = chew less = larger swallows = eat more = savor less

HOW TO DE-WOLF

Imagine those sexy pictures, commercials, and ads of a woman's mouth open to take a bite of something to be enjoyed, like a piece of succulent chocolate. I am obviously not saying your face has to be perfectly photoshopped with perfectly lined lips and white teeth. That is just ridiculous, fake, and so many things I am not willing to go into here. What I *am* saying is to bite like that woman is biting.

Her teeth are not bared with her mouth open as far as it can and her lips stretched and drawn away to take the largest bite of the dessert as she can. The woman's lips and partly-open mouth are highlighted, with just the bottom edges of her teeth visible.

My point is try eating like this. Choose a smaller fork, and focus on putting a smaller amount of food on your utensil. Then take a bite in this manner, as if you were in the ad. Practice. I know we are going against many, many years of deeply ingrained habits of chowing down as much as you can as fast as you can, but any habit can be relearned. If you try this, you will be forced to take *much* smaller bites, I promise you that.

RECAP

It's time to unlearn the habit of stuffing as much food into our mouths as possible. Use a smaller utensil. Put less food on your fork. And only put as much into your mouth as you can fit without baring your teeth like a wolf.

17

MELTING

You can't control how you feel,
but you can always choose how you act.
—MEL ROBBINS

We do not want to be "on a diet" that restricts us to the point that we know it is not sustainable for life. The goal is to find a healthy lifestyle… a healthy "diet" for the *rest* of your life. That being said, we have to—and want to—allow ourselves to indulge a little from time to time without guilt. If we don't, we will end up binging, feeling guilty and ashamed, and restrict ourselves even more, which all turns into a very nasty revolving door down a rabbit hole with little hope we will be able to pull ourselves out.

MODERATION

A key way I have found to not overdo on the sweets is to let them melt in my mouth before chewing. That's right. Anything that is able to melt that is an indulgence or otherwise unhealthy—ice cream, candy, chocolate, etc.—let the bites melt in your mouth before you chew and swallow. Keep it on your tongue—not cheeks—and move your tongue around as it's melting to allow the flavor and texture to reach your entire tongue. You will be satisfied *sooner* and therefore eat *less* of it and will enjoy it *more* because you are able to actually taste the full flavor and sweetness before you swallow.

Savoring is the essence of enjoying, and who in their right mind would choose to *not* enjoy their food? Nonsense I tell you. Yes, the whole melting process does test your patience and anticipation, but the reward is great and may just become a new habit for you.

You know those people who are always saying, *gosh, I just don't know where the time went*, or, *it's 5pm already*??

In some cases, admittingly, that is a good thing, such as in the case when you are working intensely on a project and get into a flow state of complete immersion and focus. In that kind of state, you are able to think clearly, to be in complete laser-like focus on what you are working on, and get a crap-ton done. All of a sudden, 3 hours have gone by, and you feel hugely accomplished by your focus and what you got done. That is good.

It becomes self-hurtful, however, when a habit is developed of going through life fuzzy by not fully submerging yourself and appreciating what is around you. Or as the phrase goes, taking the time to stop and smell the roses.

This same principle applies to food.

Take a bar of chocolate, for instance. Yes, you can break off a piece, put it in your mouth, chew it, taste it, and swallow. This takes approximately 5-7 seconds, and you end up swallowing pieces of chocolate and haven't really tasted *all* of the chocolate. Or you could break off a piece, put it in your mouth, and let it sit there. As it melts, the yummy gooiness spreads and fills your entire mouth.

This takes, I would surmise, 30-40 seconds... much longer for the same piece of chocolate, and yet you get that mental feel-good rush of pleasure and satisfaction from the taste much more quickly and fully than simply chewing and swallowing. As the warmth of your mouth, tongue, and saliva soften and melt the sweet treat, there will be a small explosion of flavor in your mouth.

The flavors and textures of food is one of life's pleasures, and by making yourself fully aware of them, time seems to pass more slowly because you are in the moment, thereby tricking your brain into thinking you have had much more than you really have... and yet you were able to enjoy and taste it more. So, let it melt and thoroughly enjoy that which can be melted and fill your mouth and taste buds with the rich (I'm assuming it's a dessert here) flavors.

You're welcome!

RECAP

Eat less of your desserts and sweet treats and taste them much more fully by letting the bites melt in your mouth before chewing and swallowing.

18

CHEWING

You can't stop the waves, but you can learn to surf.
—Jon Kabat-Zinn

Many of us know that one person that when he chews, it looks like he is on 2x time and should be talking like a chipmunk. You laugh, but seriously. I wonder how much he really is enjoying his food when it's chewed and swallowed within one gigasecond. I may be exaggerating a little, but I really do know a person like that.

ENJOY

My point is that while food is meant to be fuel, food is doctored up to be enjoyed and savored. Since we all enjoy food that is pleasing to our palate, why not enjoy the experience longer? The more time it takes to chew and swallow each bite, the more you taste it for a longer period of time, the more you feel you have eaten.

More time taken to eat = more time enjoying it

EAT LESS

You will eat less in the *present* because of both physiological and psychological factors. Physically, the stomach takes about 20 minutes to send the signals to your brain that you are full. Psychologically, you are tasting the yumminess for a longer period of time, which tricks your brain into thinking you had *more* of it than you actually did. This means the longer you prolong the mealtime by chewing slower, the *fuller* you will be *sooner* into your meal.

Wait, there's more. You will eat less in the *future* too. The quicker you chew and swallow, the more you overeat. We already established this. But what this *means* is you end up stretching your stomach out *before* it sends the full signals to your brain. The *more* food it will take in the future for those stretch receptors to signal your brain you are done.

Chew slower = eat less = stomach requires less food to be full

HEARTBURN

Digestion, as a whole, is the sum of many different chain reactions that start with you thinking about, seeing, and/or smelling food. That's right, your body starts preparing for the food *before* you have even taken a bite.

We all know our saliva glands start the process by excreting saliva, but what we can't feel or see is the stomach beginning to excrete more acid in preparation for the food. Not only that, but the small intestine *also* readies itself for the movement and absorption of food.

The faster we chew and get the food swallowed, the less time all of these processes have to ready the body for the food you are giving it. Your body is subsequently much less effective at breaking the food down and absorbing what it needs in order to function optimally before being passed through. Indigestion, heartburn, gas, and bloating are just some of what may follow as a result of rushing this process.

Eat fast = undigested food = tummy problems

RECAP

The longer you chew, the longer it will take for you to finish a meal, the less you will eat, the more effective you will be at avoiding weight gain.

Conversely, the faster you chew, the quicker you eat, and the more food (a.k.a. calories) you can sneak in. Before you know it, you finish the entire meal *before* your natural satiation ("full") signals kick in, and you are uncomfortably full of many more calories ingested than you need.

19

CENTERING

All life is an experiment.
The more experiments you make, the better.
—RALPH WALDO EMERSON

lvin, Simon, and Theodore... doo, doo, doodoodoodoo. One of my favorite cartoons growing up was *Alvin and the Chipmunks*. Theodore was my favorite; he was just so silly, cute, and lovable.

CUTE CHIPMUNK CHEEKS

Let's keep the cute chipmunk cheeks for the chipmunks.

We are not chipmunks. We do not need to be storing food in our cheeks, yet that is what happens when we take too large of bites. Pay attention next time you are eating... does a portion of your food get pushed to your cheeks as you are chewing the rest of the bite you just took?

If so, your bite was too large. This is a great way to monitor the size bite you take. It's one thing to say the blanket statement, take smaller bites. Well, that's great, but how big of a bite *should* I be taking?

Here's a good rule of thumb to go by: If you can keep all the food in the bite you just took in the *center* of your mouth—inside the space between your teeth—and no food has to escape to your cheeks to allow room for chewing and tasting a portion of the bite, then *that* is the bite size you should be taking.

JIPPED

If you were to eat a lunch you were looking forward to that ended up being very bland, lacked flavor, and it took you 7 minutes to eat it, you would feel jipped, like you wanted *more* to fulfill your expectations and feel satisfied. Now imagine taking 7 minutes to eat that exact same thing, but it was flavorful and exactly what you had been expecting. You would feel satiated and satisfied. Now apply this same thing to the individual bites you take.

There are many saliva glands in your cheeks. If food escapes into your cheeks as your overly-large bite of food is chewed, while the food is out there, the saliva will begin going to work on that food without you even tasting it. When it makes its way back where you can actually taste it on your tongue, it's already lost some of its flavor and texture.

TONGUE IS FOR TASTING

Your tongue is where you taste your food, not outside your teeth in your cheeks. If you keep the food—and flavor—in the center of your mouth where you can actually taste and enjoy it, you get the satisfaction from eating it. Conversely, if you take a bite too large, keep food in your cheeks, chew fast and not enough, you will be jipped of that mental satisfaction, and you will be left with wondering where the food went and why you still want more... *and* most likely get more food to feel that satisfaction.

Why is this important? The smaller bite sizes, the longer it takes to get through your meal, the sooner you feel full, the more you can taste your food, and the more pleasure you get from eating and tasting your food... *and* it lasts longer. It's a win-win situation!

Small bites = eat longer = taste more = full sooner = more pleasure

RECAP

Keep the food on top of your tongue as you chew and move it around. You will be *much* more rewarded; you will be able to thoroughly taste the food, and your brain will be able to recognize the different flavors and textures. If you are not able to prevent it from escaping to your cheeks, your bite is too large.

20

BREATHING

You may not control all the events that happen to you, but you can decide not to be reduced by them.
—MAYA ANGELOU

Pinch your nose, close your eyes, choose a jellybean, put it in your mouth. What do you taste?

Only sweetness. No flavor.

Release your nose, and suddenly you can taste the cherry or lemon flavor of the candy.

Remember being sick as a kid and having to take the disgusting-tasting liquid medicine? Remember how it didn't taste quite as bad when we pinched our noses while swallowing? Or you know how it's more difficult to taste food if our noses are stuffy from being sick?

This smelling/tasting relationship also applies to something *yummy* in your mouth. Here are four reasons why you want to keep from chomping like a dog and, instead, close your mouth and breathe through your nose:

SMELLING = MORE YUMMINESS

1— Your tongue is only responsible for the basic tastes: salty, sweet, sour, bitter, umami, and some fats. To truly "taste" and appreciate the complexity of a food's unique taste, you must keep your mouth shut while chewing and breathe through your nose. It not only allows you to inhale the aromas as you take a bite, but it also allows you to take the smells from the food *already* in your mouth into your nose as you *exhale*, thus allowing you to "taste" more richly, deeply, and complexly. The more you involve your sense of smell while eating, the more satisfaction you will have from eating, leaving you satisfied.

SALIVATION = MORE YUMMINESS

2— Your saliva glands are made to react to the type, texture, and amount of food in your mouth and secrete adequate saliva to accommodate those variables. By not opening your mouth, the food will stay moist, and saliva will circulate the flavors more fully, making for a much more delectable and satisfying bite, *every* bite. With your mouth open, your saliva glands have a harder time detecting the type, amount, and texture of the food you are eating and will secrete less, and your mouth will stay drier.

Try this—try chewing anything while not closing your lips *at all*. Notice the tastes and ease of swallowing. Now take another bite of the same type of food and the same amount and leave your lips closed the entire time while chewing and swallowing. I guarantee the flavors will be more intense as more saliva carries the food around your entire mouth. The food melts and melds together more when your mouth is kept shut.

TUMMY ISSUES

3— The air going into your nose goes to your lungs. The air going into your mouth can go to either your lungs or stomach. Keeping your mouth closed while chewing and swallowing reduces that air that gets inadvertently swallowed into your stomach. The swallowed air makes us feel bloated and uncomfortable. Who wants to have a stomach ache, feel "poufy," and have extra gas? Not me.

BE CONSIDERATE

4— People do not want to see the half-masticated food swirling around in your mouth as you chew.

RECAP

Purposefully breathing through your nose requires that your mouth be closed while chewing, forcing you to take smaller bites, eat slower, and eat less before you feel as though you are full. You will experience a heightened sense of taste and get more satisfaction out of each bite, fulfilling your cravings and desire for the food more quickly.

21

COUNTING

Count how many times I chew each bite? Are you serious?

To practice with at first, yes, I think it is a good idea. If you are having difficulty with eating too much or scarfing your food or weight control, this may help. It is a method of being mindful and paying attention to how much you are helping the digestion process along versus how much you are swallowing whole.

CRAVINGS

Listen, your body craves things when you are not fed. Meaning, when you are not getting the vitamins and nutrients your body *needs* to live, function, and survive at an optimal level, your body suffers and wants more. Let me make this as un-jargon-y and un-boring as possible...

When your body has to work harder than it otherwise should because you are not giving it the dense nutrition it needs... to do the basic functions it needs to... and to get those functions done... it takes energy from other sources... or it doesn't do those functions as well.

The result? You are drained of energy because your body is taking those resources from other places or your body has to compensate in some way.

The more you chew your food, the better your body is able to break down and absorb that food, both before *and* after you swallow it. The more it is able to break down and absorb, the more you benefit. This means the more you are absorbing and benefiting from the nutrients and vitamins, the *better* you will feel, the more *energy* you will have, and the *better* mood you will be in.

Don't forget, the more you chew your food, the longer it takes for you to finish your meal, thus allowing you to enjoy the meal longer and allowing your body to recognize it's fuller faster. In other words, you will feel better, eat less, and taste it longer... all from chewing each bite more. Who knew something so simple could do so much?

ENERGY

Have you ever felt drained or tired after finishing a meal? Did you know your chews have an effect on that? The longer you chew, the more you are breaking the food down in your mouth, the less your stomach and intestines have to work, the less energy it will take digest your food, the more energy you will feel after finishing your meal.

CALORIES

Increasing the number of times you chew your food before swallowing reduces the amount of food consumed, fewer calories are consumed, and more appetite-suppressing hormones are released that tell your brain when to stop eating. Again, a win-win.

HABIT

If you need a number to start with to get in the habit, try 30 chews per bite. If the number game isn't your thing, another way to determine if you have chewed enough to sufficiently start the digestion process is you should continue to chew your food until it loses all of its texture or until no lumps remain in your mouth. It should be almost a paste before you swallow. Gross-sounding, I know. But this requires you to remain in the present and remain aware of the food in your mouth, which will also increase satiation. May I say it again? Win, win.

TUMMY ISSUES

If that doesn't have you convinced, how about less bacteria entering your body, less bloating and gas, and less constipation and diarrhea? Starch and sugar should be pre-digested by our saliva. If we don't chew our food enough in order to let the saliva do its job, our stomach and intestines are forced to do the digesting of those types of foods it shouldn't have to do all by itself. Also, the taste buds in the mouth tell the brain what type of food we are eating to prompt the appropriate type and amount of digestive juices to begin to be released in our gut before the food even gets there. If you aren't able to thoroughly taste it because you are swallowing before it's chewed, the gut isn't ready. Want to avoid a stomach ache? Chew your food well.

RECAP

You will feel better, eat less, and taste food longer. All from chewing each bite more

22

SENSING

Grant me the strength to focus this week, to be mindful and present, to serve with excellence, to be a force of love.
—BRENDON BURCHARD, *THE CHARGE*

Our mind is like a butterfly, directed not by the wind, but by our focus. There are countless distractions, to-dos, sounds, colors, people... how can you truly, deeply focus on and enjoy one single little thing and take it all in with all of life's distractions?

CLOSE YOUR EYES

To truly taste your food is to truly realize you are eating it. If you are scarfing down your food while doing other things and while paying attention to other goings-on around you, you lose some of the satisfaction of eating the food that would otherwise be very pleasing.

Have you heard of someone who loses one of their senses, perhaps their sight, who then experiences a heightening of one of their other senses, like their hearing?

Our brain uses *all* of our senses to anticipate the enjoyment of our food. Closing your eyes seals off one of those senses while having food in the mouth. It eliminates one facet of distraction and mindlessness. Closing your eyes heightens your sense of taste as you are intensely concentrating on the food on your tongue. It allows you to depend on the other senses and fully savor the smells and flavors.

OVEREATING

Part of the reason we overeat is we feel like it went by too fast, like we didn't get to taste it, pay attention to it, or enjoy it long enough. And so we eat more to enjoy that taste and texture a little while longer.

I, of course, am not saying to eat with your eyes closed all of the time. You would definitely get some odd looks in a restaurant, for sure. But I *am* saying that when you feel comfortable, perhaps while eating alone, give it a try, and see how much more you *actually* taste your food.

It won't take *all* distraction out of course, because you still have all of your other senses, but it will take the sense of sight out of the equation.

RECAP

Try chewing with your eyes closed. This will heighten your sense of taste and allow you to practice fully concentrating and appreciating the food you are eating.

Restaurants: you may get looked at funny.
Home: the most ideal spot.

23

SWALLOWING

We can't solve problems by using the same kind of thinking we used when we created them.
—ALBERT EINSTEIN

When eating with friends or family or when out at a restaurant, there is little else that is worse than watching a person shovel food in his mouth and subsequently seeing the half-chewed, saliva-drenched food still in his mouth as he opens wide for another bite. It makes me gag just imagining it.

*SEE*FOOD WITH A SIDE OF *GAG*ME

Not only is it disgusting to see, but a conveyor-belt type of eating naturally produces a faster eating experience with a generous side of overeating.

Why would you *not* want to taste your food and enjoy it *all* before taking another bite? What is the function served by repeatedly shoveling in food before you are done chewing and swallowing what is already in your mouth?

I don't think I'll ever know, but I am telling you from the health side of it, it results in you eating faster—obviously since the mouth is never completely empty—which also makes you eat more. Your body needs time to recognize how much you have eaten and if, and when, you are full. Until a certain amount of time has passed—about 20 minutes until your "reaching capacity" brain signals kick in—we can shovel *a lot* in before that if we eat in this manner.

Swallow each bite = eat slower = eat less

NOT A RACE

Eating is not a race. I understand there are seasons of life that force you to be "trained" to eat quickly. For instance, those in the military must eat quickly. Or as a kid, you learned to eat quickly before your siblings took your food.

You picked up this book for a reason, and I am assuming it was to learn how to change a bad eating habit that is not serving you in your current life. The lovely part of the being "trained" to eat quickly at one point in your life also means you can be "*un*trained." It may take some work, some practice, some trial and error, just as it did while you were learning to eat quickly, but you *can* undo that bad habit. The portions will *still* be there on your plate when you get to them, whether it is in 2 minutes or 10 minutes. The only reason I can possibly see to scarfing your food down by taking bites before you are done chewing and swallowing is if you are worried about it getting cold. Think of it this way: the food will get cold within the same amount of time whether it's half the plate full or the whole plate full. You may as well slow it down and eat half as much in the same amount of time.

You have a choice. You can go slower and eat half the plate's worth in that amount of time, being able to savor and actually taste the food and eat less of it … *or* … shovel it *all* in in the same amount of time, forkful by forkful, swallowing partial large lumps to make room for the next forkful, not really tasting it, not letting the flavors and richness of the food permeate your entire mouth, and not allowing you to fully enjoy it.

Let's do ourselves a favor and do everyone else eating with you a favor. Enjoy your food, and allow the people with you to enjoy theirs as well. Let's agree to concentrate on practicing chewing and swallowing *all* of the food in our mouths before taking another bite… or talking.

RECAP

Swallow all of your food in your mouth before you open your mouth to take another bite. It allows you to taste and savor more of your food, as well as eat slower and eat less.

24

SEPARATING

By doing what you would do if you were exactly the person you'd like to be, you'll ultimately become that person.
—BRIAN TRACY

I have been guilty of many things related to bad eating habits, including taking huge bites, inhaling my food, caving to my cravings... and every once in a while, I'll be in such a rush I will mindlessly take a sip of liquid while food is still in my mouth to get it down faster. My first thought immediately is, *Eww.*

I have noticed a legitimate reason for the mixing of food and drink is if the food is unexpectantly too hot either in temperature or spiciness. However, the manner by which it becomes a habit stumps me. Aren't foods usually eaten to enjoy their flavor and/or texture? It baffles me why someone would develop the habit of creating a mangled mush of nothingness in their mouth.

IN A HURRY

It seems the main reason is to hurry along the chewing and swallowing process... almost like their saliva glands are not moistening their bites in time with the pace at which they wish to eat and swallow their food.

Well then, why not just pour your water directly onto your plate of food; it would make the process even faster by not having to pause to take a drink with every bite.

Yes, I am being sarcastic. Regardless of the reason, if you engage in this sort of eating, however infrequently, try refraining from this practice. You get very little enjoyment from the flavor of food when it is mixed with whatever beverage you are having with your meal, leaving you feeling unsatisfied and wanting more. Not only that but, sorry to say, people don't want to see your half-masticated food as you open your mouth to take the drink.

If this is you, you are rushing the eating process way too much and robbing yourself of the pleasure of both the food and the beverage you have chosen for your meal. If you can't wait to naturally have your saliva do its thing, then you are either waiting too long before you eat and starving yourself, or you are being too impatient, or both.

RECAP

Chew your food, taste your food, swallow your food, and *then* take the drink. Do not combine the food and drink together in your mouth.

25

SHOVELING

Through discipline comes freedom.
—ARISTOTLE

Food is meant to be enjoyed, especially when you are in the company of other people. Being the first one done should not be the goal and is not an accomplishment. Eating is not an inconvenience or intrusion to be gotten through as soon as possible.

Many of us—myself included—sometimes go into conveyor-belt-mode by automatically filling the utensil immediately when it's empty while still chewing. To do so creates an unnecessary sense of urgency, which prompts you to chew faster and swallow before you should… all in the name of doing *something* with that forkful of food in your hand staring you in the face.

In addition to not giving yourself the time to taste your food, scarfing down the food in 5 minutes in conveyor-belt-like fashion does not give you the opportunity to reflect on your fullness when the next bite is always waiting for you. The tendency then is to eat until there is nothing left to eat, especially since those hormone signals of satiety and fullness aren't activated until it's too late and you're on your 10th cookie. You're feeling out of control, and over time, eventual weight gain is pretty much guaranteed.

ONE OF LIFE'S PLEASURES

Despite what you may have told yourself, food is meant to be enjoyed and savored. *Actually* pay attention to how much you rush chewing and swallowing when you have food already on your fork waiting for you to swallow. And pay attention to the unswallowed food you still have in your cheeks or in the back of your throat as you take that next bite.

When you are able, take the time and halt the conveyor belt. Resist the urge to shovel it in, bite after half-eaten bite.

While you are chewing the bite you just put in your mouth, keep your utensil empty while you are still chewing. Bonus points if you put your utensil down after each few bites. This is true for finger foods as well, such as sandwiches, raw vegetables, french fries, etc. Put the food down on the plate after a few bites. Mega bonus points if it is after each bite. You will focus more on the flavor and texture of the food in your mouth in that moment rather than thinking about and anticipating the next.

RECAP

Eating is not a contest. Put down your utensil between bites and take smaller forkfuls. The more time you take to eat, the fewer calories you will consume.

26

INTERMISSION

Don't be pushed around by the fears in your mind.
Be led by the dreams in your heart.
—ROY T BENNETT

Mind over matter. No this isn't the movies or a play. It's a meal, and you *can* take an "intermission" in the middle of eating a meal. This is a trick I use quite often, especially when I notice myself eating too quickly at the beginning. For me, that usually happens when we are out, and I am super excited about the yummy food in front of me. It's just so stinking good that I dive right in, taking large bites, swallowing quickly… well, you know the drill. I soon realize it, set my fork down, and remember that I want to *taste* it and *enjoy* it, and I remind myself that I do not need to eat everything in front of me.

This "intermission" resets my focus and intentions, allowing me to be more present when I do continue eating. It *also* let's my brain catch up with my stomach and how full it *actually* is. But at what point do you take the intermission, and let the food settle before continuing to eat?

OPTION 1: HALVES IT

You have two options. 1— Before you begin to eat the food on your plate, divide it in half. 2— Or only take half as much as you would normally put on your plate (this would also help the rest stay warm).

Whichever method you choose, it can be either done mentally or actually divide it out on your plate. The latter is preferred since it gives you a clearly defined point at which to stop. Also, you will be less likely to convince yourself to eat more if you can actually *see* the point at which you will intend to take the intermission.

Be sure to decide in advance how long your intermission will be. I recommend at least 2-3 minutes, but 5-7 minutes is ideal. I know the 5-7 minutes is unrealistic if you are out to eat or eating at work. However, if you are eating while watching TV or you are in otherwise not a huge rush, it *is* possible to do.

Eat one half of your meal, and when you are done with that half, put your fork down, and start sipping on water while you engage in what is going on around you, whether it is admiring the view, eavesdropping on the next table's conversation, watching the show you are watching, or fully engaging in the conversation going on at your own table.

OPTION 2: FOURTHS IT

Another option is to take 3-4 mini-breaks throughout the meal of 1-2 minutes each. This is the less noticeable option when eating out with friends. Engage in conversation with the people with you, look around at your surroundings, sit back in your chair and make circles with your feet... I don't care. Just slow it down.

WATER

Whichever method you choose, be sure you are sipping consistently on water throughout this intermission time. The goal is to drink a full 8 ounces of water by the time you pick your fork back up and resume eating the other half of your meal... if you can even fit it. I guarantee you, though, you will feel less hungry and thereby eat less once you resume. This is a great method to stay in control and not be at the mercy of your cravings, your desires, or your appetite.

RECAP

Take time during your meals to set your food down, and sip on water. You most likely will eat less when you resume eating than you would have if you had not divided your food, not taken an intermission, and just continued eating.

27

DAYDREAMING

*You are the designer of your destiny;
you are the author of your story.*
—LISA NICHOLS

When you are eating for any other reason besides actual, real hunger—whether out of boredom, or emotions, or a few adult beverages—and you have chosen something that you feel a little guilty or bad about, it's easier to deal with that guilt or shame by *not* feeling it, right? And you check out a little, almost like your mind gets a little fuzzy or cloudy. This is a common defense mechanism we use during a bad situation to delay having to mentally deal with it. It's a way to get through the bad times, basically.

Number 1— You shouldn't be feeling guilty about anything you put in your mouth, because if you are, that means one of two things… 1— you are on a "diet" that is restricting you, or 2— you have lost control over your eating. Both of which needs to be addressed in order for the guilt, shame, and mind cloudiness to be lifted.

Number 2— If you are able to stay in the moment, feeling every texture of your food, tasting every taste, and savoring it, you will eat less of it. Haven't you ever started mindlessly snacking, and before you know it, a whole row of Oreos is gone? And you think, well gosh, I know I ate them, but I don't really *remember* tasting all of them. If you would have been in the present, tasting and savoring every Oreo, you most likely would have had only 3 or 4... or 6. Probably not the whole 12.

When you are not present, it is easier to eat compulsively or binge-eat and then feel ashamed, regretful, and out of control. It is similar to having your name called when you are lost in thought. You immediately snap out of your daydream. The goal here is to never enter the daydream in the first place while you are eating but to stay present, focused, and aware. If you realize you are getting all fuzzy-brained, put down your utensil or food, and take a minute to refocus on how your body feels and the food you are giving it.

This is *not* about restricting or punishing. This *is* about allowing yourself grace and allowing yourself treats, but in moderation. All in moderation. And moderation is much, much easier achieved if you remain present in the moment and aware of each bite.

RECAP

Stay present with each bite, and you will likely eat less of it, especially if it is a treat.

28

SAVORING

Rule your mind, or it will rule you.
—BUDDHA

For me, it's pizza and doughnuts. What is it for you? What is it that you tend to crave when you do crave things? What is it that you consider a real treat because you find it *that* yummy and satisfying? For many people, it is a sweet treat of some kind. Other people crave more of the salty or greasy kinds of foods. I am usually more of the salty kind of girl.

How can you tell when a certain food is your downfall or nemesis? Do you usually mindlessly eat it? Do you reach for it when you are bored, depressed, stressed, anxious, or lonely? Do you feel guilt or shame after you have eaten it?

NEGOTIATE AHEAD OF TIME

If you are going to have and sustain a healthy attitude toward food for the long-haul, you have to tell yourself that *no* food is *completely* off-limits *all* of the time. Feeling deprived and depressed is not the goal here.

Allow me to explain.

You are at a party. You like carrots. You love chocolate. If you have the option of chocolate or carrots at a party, and you tell yourself you cannot have the chocolate and opt for the carrots with absolutely no chocolate, first—kudos to you for your willpower and dedication, but second—*please* do not do that. Yes, you heard me right. By making the chocolate a "forbidden fruit," you are putting it on a pedestal and placing far more value on it than the carrots that now have less value.

Instead, negotiate with yourself. Set an amount of *both* to have *before* taking any of it. You are thus allowing yourself both and enjoying them both for different reasons but with the same value and on a level playing field.

GUILT-FREE MODERATION

If you feel deprived, you are dieting, and we don't want to diet; we want a sustainable, healthy lifestyle we can build a foundation on for the rest of our lives. Yes, there will be "bad" nights of too many cocktails, desserts, fried foods, and all out fun. Yes, there will "bad" weekends, bad weeks, and even bad months. But this foundation of a healthy mindset, healthy habits, and a healthful palate will carry us and always bring us back. None of us are perfect, and when you stop expecting yourself to be, you are able to release the guilt-chains that are choking you.

Here is how to have your cake and eat it too (Literally!)... but in moderation:

1. Take a bite the size a child would take.
2. Keep your mouth closed.

3. Let it sit on your tongue to melt slightly as saliva fills your mouth and carries the taste you are craving to all parts of your mouth.
4. Chew slowly.
5. Roll the bite around your mouth with your tongue as you chew.
6. Close your eyes and fully focus on the yumminess.
7. Chew it until very small and very broken down.
8. Swallow.

DOWNFALL = ASSET

Your greatest temptation or that food (or foods) you love to hate that you love but your body hates (follow that?) is really a great asset to you.

Why?

Because you get to practice with it. Practice everything we have learned in this section with that food. So yes, I am telling you to go out and buy that.

Say what?!?

Yes, bring it into your house. Buy it *un*-economically, as we discussed in a previous chapter, and in small quantities, but I *am* giving you guilt-free permission to spend your hard-earned money on an indulgence that is probably not welcome in your body.

Why?

So you can see what I mean about savoring... about being in the moment... about being present... about control... about eating less of it but still enjoying it the same as if you had a huge amount of it... about staying guilt-free with the bad stuff even though it is bad stuff.

RECAP

Buy your downfall in small, un-economical quantities, and practice the art of savoring it, as detailed above

29

OVEREATING

*Don't make a habit out of choosing what feels good
over what's actually good for you.*
—Eric Thomas

When I go to a favorite restaurant of mine and order an awesome dinner salad, gosh I just feel so confident and in control. I just made the healthy choice when I really wanted the cheeseburger and fries. I didn't feel bad about eating the entire thing *and* my husband's breadsticks because I just had a salad for dinner, for gosh sakes. Woohoo! Bring on the extra drink since I deserve it for making the healthy choice. Dessert anyone?

Sound familiar?

Did you know you can overeat healthy food also? For instance, you think you are doing the healthy thing by ordering the Southwestern Salad with grilled chicken from a popular sit-down chain restaurant. You even get it without the croutons and with the dressing on the side. That's called a win, right? Gosh, I would love to think so because I love salad and could use as many mental wins as possible, but unfortunately that is not always the case, especially if you finish the entire salad.

If you knew that salad alone was 1010 calories, would you eat the entire thing? Or even order it at all when most of their other chicken dishes are under 700 calories? Add on two of their breadsticks to that salad and an innocent glass of wine, and you are looking at 1540 calories. It is a huge salad with a ton of stuff added to it to, yes you guessed it, make it tasty. All of sudden you just overate big time on what is widely accepted the healthy choice.

I just want you to be aware that a healthy choice doesn't mean you have free-reign to eat as much as you want without consequence. The consequence may not be that night because all of the ingredients *seemed* real and raw, and one unhealthy, very large meal won't make you "fat," but consistently over time eating this way will end you in trouble. The compound effect will take place. And all of a sudden, a year later, you are as confused as ever because you have been "eating healthy" and actually *gained* weight and feel terrible. You decide this healthy eating for the lifespan is just "not for you" and doesn't "work for you," so you do a crash diet or fad diet and start the inevitable cycling of yo-yo dieting and not sustaining anything you want.

RECAP

The lesson? Apply all of the tips, tricks, and tactics in this book to the "healthy" food as well. Feeling like you have free reign on healthy foods, especially healthy foods that are pre-made for you, is dangerous.

If you obey all the rules, you miss all the fun.
—KATHERINE HEPBURN

AFTER PARTY

A pessimist sees the difficulty in every opportunity.
An optimist sees the opportunity in every difficulty.
—WINSTON CHURCHILL

30

JOURNALING

I would suggest keeping a food journal for a period of 7 days so it spans both your workweek and your weekend. If you do not have a set schedule, such as you are on-call, 7 days is long enough to give you an average estimate of what you are consuming. During these 7 days, eat as you normally would, grabbing the handful of candy as you walk by the secretary's desk, drinking the normal sodas and juices you normally do.

Journaling everything that passes through your mouth allows you to track and figure out exactly how much you really are eating and which ones make you feel like crap and which ones makes you feel energized, which ones make you feel like taking a nap and which ones support your workout, which ones make you gain weight and which ones support your weight loss (as long as you are weighing yourself every day when you wake up).

A journal furthermore makes you keenly aware as you go through your day what exactly you are eating that you may not even remember, like the mindless handful of M&M'S® you grab as you walk by the secretary's desk. If you typically have your smart phone with you, as most people now do, recording this in an application—or "app"—is a much quicker and more convenient method to record your intake. Put this app on your home screen, on the first page, so you don't even have to swipe right or left.

If you prefer the paper version, you then must find a way to keep it with you at all times during this 7-day trial. Don't rely on memory; it fails us all the time. Whether it be a purse big enough in which to carry it or to look for a journal small enough to fit in your pocket. There are small 2"x 3" notepads that are about the size of a man's wallet available at just about any store that carries office supplies of any kind.

There are many versions of paper food journals, as well as many versions of apps, available to suit your preferences and needs. You may have to do a little researching—or "Google it" as I call it—to find the right one for you. There are even journals you can download off the internet to your phone or to print. Often times having that perfect app with just the right features or a journal with just the right prompts can be what makes the difference in providing the interest and motivation to commit to it. Don't be afraid to try a few different ones. And don't automatically forego the apps or journals that you have to pay for; exchanging a few dollars for the journal or app gives you "skin in the game," which may prompt you to carry through with it and utilize it more than if it were a free journal.

RECAP

Keep a food journal to track what and how much you are eating and drinking.

31

ADAPTING

I never lose. Either I win, or I learn.
—UNKNOWN

ailure will happen. Just expect the mess-ups. But giving the mess-ups too much credit and focus can lead us to eat... a lot... of the bad stuff. Your perspective and reaction, however, to that "failure" makes *all* the difference. I want you to check your expectation of perfection at the door and let in the grace and forgiveness you deserve.

EXPECT AND ADAPT

You are going to eat and drink too much of the wrong thing at the wrong time. You are going to mess up—a lot. Everyone does. Life is all about the learning curve. If you are not failing at things, you are not even trying, and therefore things will never change. So expect a failure here and there. Expect the weight fluctuations here and there. Expect the hangovers, bloat, stomach aches, etc. Look forward to this which I call the "adjustment phase;" it means you get to become that much more of an expert about your own body that is always changing, always adapting, and always working.

Learning and enjoying a clean eating lifestyle without the limits of a restricting "diet" takes trial and error. Learn from it, adjust, and continue. Know that each "mistake," as long as you reflect on it and how you feel after, is teaching you and molding you to a better you tomorrow.

NO PUNISHMENTS

Do not—ever—"punish" yourself for losing control and eating too much of the wrong thing, whether it's by restricting yourself the next day or week or with exercise or anything else. Do this, and you will start to associate both indulging and healthy eating with something bad. This starts a very negative downward spiral that eventually impacts your behaviors, habits, and attitude toward this whole thing.

Instead, plan for the following day while still allowing the treats in moderation—how will you get back on track tomorrow without starving yourself or cardio-ing yourself to death? What will that look like? How will you feel about yourself after a good day of having full control over your eating again? Establish some non-food rewards for yourself to help keep you moving forward. It's a choice to keep going, to keep adjusting, to keep learning, and to keep staying positive. You are *brave* and *amazing*.

RECAP

Perfection is an illusion, so drop that expectation. Never punish. Reflect, learn, adapt, plan, and rock it tomorrow.

32

CLOSING

Create on purpose instead of by default.
—MELISSA PHARR

The time we spend with the people we love is often centered in the kitchen or around food. Gathering in that room and continuing with the snacking and drinking caloric beverages late into the night is common for many families. And sometimes we are in a busy and unpredictable season of life that keeps us up late at night.

If your schedule allows, have a kitchen shut-down time to give your stomach and digestive system a rest. That means after that time, there is no more snacking—even if it's just air-popped popcorn—and no drinking other than water.

Determining, agreeing on, and setting this time *with* your roommate, spouse, kids, or family as a whole can be an important step to prevent resentment toward this new standard of living. A safe rule of thumb is to shut down the eating and drinking everything except water 2 hours before you go to sleep.

BENEFITS

Your body needs to focus on the processes that happen during your sleeping hours, like repairing muscles and preparing your body for your day tomorrow. Having to digest a lot of food, some of which may be more difficult if it has a lot of artificial ingredients, causes you to store more fat, have more difficulty with weight control, not sleep as well, and have heartburn and indigestion. Your body needs to heal and recharge during the night, not digest and distribute food and nutrients. It's a simple solution to better sleep quality, better weight control, and fewer tummy issues.

RECAP

Set a time at which your home kitchen is closed, meaning no more food or beverages other than pure water after a certain time.

33

SLEEPING

We all get what we tolerate. Stop tolerating excuses within yourself, limiting beliefs of the past, and half-assed or fearful states.
—TONY ROBBINS

I know sleep sounds unrelated to hunger, eating, and cravings. But it is not, and let me explain why before you skip over this chapter. The more you know the reasoning behind what actually happens, the more apt you will be to take the steps necessary to get the sleep you need.

SLEEP'S POWERS

It takes your brain about 20 minutes to get the signals from the stretch receptors in your stomach that your stomach is full enough. Before then, there is a hormone, Ghrelin, produced in your stomach that reminds the pleasure centers in your brain of how yummy those cookies are and has you reaching for more. Ghrelin is *increased* when you are sleep-deprived.

In other words, get more sleep to help have fewer cravings and more willpower and discipline.

Have you ever noticed you crave sweets and carbs *more* when you are tired? It is not only your mentality that is compromised, it is your biology as well. Your body recognizes when you have not had enough sleep and are 'dragging.' Your body knows when you do not have enough energy to supply the level of activity at which you are typically performing.

Your body then tells your mind you need more energy now. What foods give your cells and muscles the most cellular energy the fastest? You guessed it—simple carbs and sugars. You not getting enough sleep leads to cravings of some of the worst foods for your waistline and overall health and vitality.

RECAP

Want fewer bad-foods cravings? Do yourself a favor, and go to bed earlier.

I can do everything through Him who gives me strength.
—PHILIPPIANS 4:13

EXTRAS

Inspiration exists, but it has to find you working.
—PABLO PICASSO

34

BOTTLING

By failing to prepare, you are preparing to fail.
—BENJAMIN FRANKLIN

We all know we need to drink more water, but a vast majority of us are mildly dehydrated. And unless we are feeling thirsty—which doesn't happen until we move into moderately dehydrated—most of us don't feel anything, especially if we are used to how we feel operating in a mildly dehydrated state day in and day out.

The absolute minimum amount of water you need to properly sustain a sedentary lifestyle is half your body weight in ounces. I'm talking a no exercise, desk job, play video games type of person. Water intake goes up to a minimum of 75% of your body weight in ounces when you are active.

NO GUESSWORK

With food, many times you have no control how the ingredients or foods themselves are processed or made. How the hidden ingredients affect your body and its functioning is often unknown and is left up to the manufacturers of the ingredients.

However, there is no guesswork with water and how it affects you. Water is easy. You know it helps your body tremendously. It's pure and organic. You know what's in it. You can control how much of it you drink, which makes this one easy way to take as much control over that aspect of your health as possible.

IMPROVE WELLBEING

Water and lots of it is the first recommended step if your goal is to lose weight, to become healthy, and/or to energize yourself. Being hydrated is pivotal in bettering your sleep, reducing the bloating (yes, if you are bloated, drink *extra* water), recovering from physical activity and exercise, improving energy and focus, transporting the good components of your food to the organs that need them, and many other positive things.

CRAVINGS

Many times, having a craving for a food is actually a function of dehydration, even if there isn't the tell-tale sign of a dry mouth. When you are dehydrated, your body knows it needs extra energy to sustain your typical level of mental and physical activity. What gives your body energy? Carbohydrates. What kind of carbs give it to you the fastest? The kind that are bad for you. Sugar. White bread and pasta. Enter cravings.

One rule of thumb to *always* go by and to adapt into your life: chug a large glass of water right when you wake up and before every meal and snack. This does not include the sugar-infused sodas, teas, coffees, or juices—instead, pure water. You will eat less and function smoother.

EAT LESS

In addition to crushing your cravings and misinterpreted "hunger," water induces a feeling of fullness. The stretch receptors in the stomach are activated by not only food but *water* as well. These receptors connect the stomach and the brain and relay the feeling of fullness. In short, drinking more water equals eating less.

PROBLEMS

Admittingly, remembering and getting enough water in during the day is difficult, especially if you're not used to it when you don't feel the physical symptom of thirst.

A method I have adopted is to always carry a typical plastic, disposable 16.9-ounce water bottle and refill it during the day. This works great when you are beginning to incorporate more water; however, now that I am used to drinking more water throughout the day, there are two problems I have encountered:

> Problem 1— Tracking the ounces during the day keeps me much more cognizant of my water intake, thus helping me to remember to chug more frequently. The problem is I sometimes lose track of how many times I fill it, or I forget to track when I get busy, running errands, or transitioning between places. Sometimes, I just have a bad day and just don't care enough that day, even though I know how important it is.

> Problem 2— Refilling the bottle before it is empty, so I'm going through the bottles but not drinking all the water. This results in an overestimation of my water intake.

SOLUTION

A great solution for all of these barriers is to purchase four larger water containers—25- or 30-ouncers. Every morning fill all four bottles up. Your goal is to get through all four bottles by the end of the day. This easily eliminates the need to remember, track, or keep count. Of course, the number and size of the bottles can and should be modified to what your body requires based on your weight and activity level, but it just makes it so easy to not have to think about or remember anything, saving brainpower for more important things. When I'm done with the bottles, I know I have had enough for the day. Easy peasy.

YOUR CHALLENGE

To be *fully* hydrated for several days in a row makes you feel… different. You feel lighter… more energetic… more alert… and you actually start craving water all the time—not just when you are "thirsty." Your mouth feels like it should have water, even though you just took a gulp 10 minutes ago and the 'old you' went hours between gulps of water. Just try it.

I challenge you! Commit to 3 days of drinking your *full* body weight in water. I recommend you do so in the middle of the work week, so for most of you, that would be Tuesday, Wednesday, Thursday— which tends to mirror what your 'typical,' most routine-filled days are like.

Post about it on Facebook or Instagram and include the hashtag **"#EatLessEnjoyMoreWaterChallenge"** when you start and when you finish the pure water challenge. At the end of every month, I randomly select one person who has done the challenge and reward that person with a $5 gift card for Amazon.

RECAP

A great solution is fill bottles every morning to be consumed by the end of the day. Take the water challenge, post about it and use the hashtag **#EatLessEnjoyMoreWaterChallenge** in Facebook or Instagram to be entered for a chance to win.

35

SUGARING

Incredible change happens in your life when you decide to take control of what you do have power over instead of craving control over what you don't.
—STEVE MARABOLI

Did you know sugar is addictive? There are two facets to this fascinating additive.

The first facet is in regard to biology and your body. Studies have shown it is more addictive than cocaine. It's no wonder then that the more you have it, the more you crave it. Your body takes on legitimate withdrawal symptoms when your body is used to it and then deprived of it. Sugar headaches, irritability, fatigue, muscle aches, cravings are just some of those symptoms. Which begs the question: do you really want to keep giving your body so much of something it becomes dependent on it?

The second facet is in regard to psychology and your taste buds. The more your taste buds are accustomed to sweet foods, the less it tastes it because it is used to it. This is why someone who rarely drinks sugary drinks or eats desserts thinks soda is overly sweet and why someone who eats and drinks sugar regularly views the sweetness of soda normal and finds plain water bland.

> *Physical: The more you eat it, the more you crave it.*
> *Psychological: The more you taste it, the more you want it.*

The key is to open your mind to the possibility that how you taste things and your opinion of them based on their taste *can* be altered for both the better *and* the worse.

HIDDEN SUGARS VS BLATANT SUGAR

Added, hidden sugars are bad, yes. Being knowledgeable and up-to-date on which foods have those sneaky, pesky sugars—like ketchup—is super important. I absolutely, 100% agree. But we are working on psychological cravings, mindset, and taste alignment. With that in mind, let's focus on the sugary *tasting* foods and how to defeat the need-more-sweetness monster.

There are two ways to gain control over your psychological need for sugary-tasting foods and drinks. The first is to go on a 3-, 5-, or 7-day sugar fast to reset and recalibrate your body and taste buds. The second is to go on a depleting system of slowly decreasing the amount of sugary drinks and foods.

> *Easier on your body: The depletion schedule.*
> *Easier on your mind: The cold-turkey approach.*

MY RECOMMENDATION

To know how much to deplete over a given time frame and to consistently reduce and refrain at specified time intervals assumes your sugar intake is consistent and requires knowing how much and how often you consume sugary-tasting drinks and foods... a.k.a. a baseline of your sugary food intake. But how do you gauge or measure sweetness? Especially if you do not bake or mix it yourself.

Yes, you can say you have dessert every night after dinner, and by knowing this, you can set the guideline to only consume half of what you would normally. But without cutting it out completely for a specified number of days, how can you definitively say you are having less without compensating for that sweetness another time of the day or in another way? Also, say you have Oreos after dinner. Do you eat the same number of Oreos every single night? Usually not.

For instance, you may know that you usually have about 6-8 cookies after dinner, and you purposefully drop it down to four. Good for you! I mean it! Have you considered, though, the extra syrup you put on your pancakes the following morning to compensate without even knowing it? Or the slightly larger piece of cake you cut at the employee appreciation lunch because unconsciously you knew your dinner dessert is less than you normally have. Or the extra-large handful of candies (when your norm is only a large handful) you mindlessly snagged out the secretary's community bowl?

There is just *a lot* of grey area that is up for discussion with the depletion method. If you are serious about getting control of this, you need a consistent *something* you have control over. Something a stranger off the street can come in and say, "Okay it is perfectly clear to me that you are indeed consuming *fewer* sugary foods *less* often during *every* day, because I can clearly see where you began and where you are now."

After a lot of thought and reflection, I just do not see how that is possible. There is just too much ambiguity.

The absolute best way is to cut it out completely for a set, short period of time to reset your mindset, perspective, and accustomed taste. As mentioned before, reintroduce sweetness slowly after that specified period of time.

You can do this. This is important. If you feel like you can't quite do this alone, unsure of how, or just need some accountability, contact me: <u>RachelZentzReaders@gmail.com</u> . I would love to help you through this.

RECAP

If you are a fan of the sweets, cut them out completely to recalibrate your taste preferences. Don't worry, it's just for a short time, then you can reintroduce sweet tasting foods and drinks in small amounts. Trust me, you'll notice a difference.

36

SALTING

My mission in life is not merely to survive, but to thrive.
—MAYA ANGELOU

A h the salty, greasy, comforting foods. They can be deep-fried, pan-fried, or just fatty meats, doesn't matter. These are my kind of foods... or they *were*. These were the ones I craved. All the way through college and into the first couple of years into my career as a school psychologist, when I was hungry and on-the-go, I didn't have a cereal bar in my purse or some nuts or a piece of fruit. And frankly, I didn't care.

My solution back then was to stop at the first fast food place I came upon and order a burger or chicken sandwich off the dollar menu. That is what I *craved*. It always came to $1.05 in Wisconsin, including tax. I knew what I liked on all of the dollar menus at all of the popular fast food chains. It always cured my hunger, cured my cravings, and cured my longing. Little did I know I was not drinking enough water and not giving my body deep nutrition that it craved.

GREASY GOODNESS

Grease, butter, and oil are common ways restaurants add flavor to foods. For instance, what typically is thought of a "good" french fry, besides the preferred level of crispiness (achieved through grease by the way), is the taste of the oil used and the type and amount of salt used. A potato is a potato; it is the *oil* that gives it its flavor that we have learned to rely on as a determining factor in its tastiness.

The more grease and flavor provided by the oil and salt, the more we crave it and expect it... and the more our taste buds become accustomed to not only it's taste but also the film ("after-taste") it leaves in your mouth long after it's swallowed, allowing us to not forget the taste of the grease we just consumed.

It is all a factor of what we *expect*... what we are *used* to... what we most often eat. If you train your taste buds (take a "break" from butter, oil, and grease) to not expect and thereby crave that type of flavoring, I promise you, you will not even miss it. Take it from a revived fast-food-aholic. The "break" will get you used to *not* expecting those flavors and tastes. Think of a good turkey chili... it achieves its depth of flavor with herbs and spices, not grease, oil, and butter.

SALT

Here was my experience; maybe you can relate... The more heavily-salted food I ate, the more I became *accustomed* to having them, the more I *wanted* them, and the more I felt foods without those salty seasonings were pretty bland and unfulfilling. The more I ate those "bland-tasting" foods with my salt-accustomed mouth, the less satiated and satisfied I felt. I just wanted something with the salty flavor I was used to. I would then overeat by indulging in that craving even after consuming and filling up on "bland-tasting" foods.

Yes, I can simply tell you to switch out your regular table salt for the healthier sea salt, but you're still getting your salty fix. The healthier salt does nothing for what your taste buds are used to or for your avoidance of "bland," simple foods (like vegetables).

The goal is to lower your *threshold*—or palate accustomedness—for salt. When this happens, you will appreciate the un-salted flavors of the simple foods more and will more likely choose these healthy alternatives. You will be more satisfied by them. And your cravings for foods high in salt (incidentally most fast food items) will diminish.

GOING INTO REHAB

You can cure this palate-addiction in one of two ways:

Option A— Cut it out completely for three days. The benefit to this is you know exactly what is expected; you simply do not reach for the salt to flavor your food. And substituting sodium-rich foods during these three days is not the option either. Pair lean proteins (no pork or red meat) with lots of veggies and limited healthy fats and fruits. No take-out or eating out of any kind.

Option B— Cut it out gradually. I personally do not favor this option because how do you know how much to cut back each day or each week when everyone is starting at a different place of salt-usage to begin with? It's not a one-size-fits-all solution in my book. Most people do not begin knowing how much salt they flavor their food with at the dinner table. I have never witnessed anyone take out the measuring spoon once the food is already cooked and on their plate. Additionally, most people do not salt all foods with the same amount of salt. My point is, if you don't know where you begin with salt intake, how do you know how much to cut if you do it gradually?

Unfortunately, I cannot be the one to tell you which would work best for you. Only you know you best. I know I can recommend and personally prefer option A for two reasons.

1— It is a very black-and-white option. There is no guessing, no room for interpretation, fudging, or cheating. It's you either use salt, or you don't. And this option is you don't. Period. Yes, your food will taste exceptionally bland the first two days. I say this from experience; I have used this method four times to reset my palate and get rid of the bloat. After the third day, though, you are golden.

2— You know your efforts are having an effect because you most likely will be craving or at the very least wishing you had the salt on the food you are eating.

In my opinion, there is too much wiggle room in option B. Go big or go home. Opt for option A, and cut it out completely. It is only three days. Quit complaining, just do it, and get it under control. It's a great way to reset those salty taste buds that by the end of the three days, you will barely want any at all.

RECAP

The more you are accustomed to salt and grease, the more you are going to crave them and the more you will eat, even after filling up on the "bland-tasting" foods. Try taking a 3-day fast from the grease and salt to recalibrate your taste buds, and get your cravings and bloat under control

It doesn't matter where you are coming from.
All that matters is where you are going.
—BRIAN TRACY

BONUS CHAPTERS

With the new day comes new strength and new thoughts.
—ELEANOR ROOSEVELT

Allow me to preface these chapters with my intentions.

The goal of this book was at first to be a collection of all of my tricks, tips, and tactics that I, being the psychologist that I am, have analyzed about myself. In all honesty, I was about 75% done with the book before I reflected on the overall theme of eating less and enjoying more. Before that theme came to fruition, I already had the following three chapters in my outline; I *knew* I wanted to debunk the hype around "diet," "all-natural," and "low fat" foods and drinks.

When I ask someone I am coaching, "What have you tried in the past?" and get the response, "I switched from regular soda to diet," I just want to reach through the computer screen or phone and shake them.

It is not only the fact that there is misperception about labeling and what it really means, but the allowances we give themselves because of the perceived "sacrifices" we are making by using to the "healthier" options is often *more* damaging.

Additionally, when you feel like you are excelling or sacrificing in one area of your life, it is human nature to allow a little more give in other areas. For instance, "*I ate healthy last night for dinner, so it's okay to stop my workout early today because I feel tired.*" Or, "*I only had two pieces of pizza instead of my usual four, so I'm going to have extra ice cream.*"

We play these mind games with ourselves all. the. time.

While these next three chapters are not directly or overtly related to eating less, indirectly and covertly they most certainly are.

37

"ALL NATURAL"

Create on purpose instead of by default.
—Melissa Pharr

We have every intention of making good decisions when it comes to spending our hard-earned money on food and drinks to feed ourselves and our families. We rely on labels and marketing to help us make those decisions to purchase the products we feel are healthy and safe and are produced and sourced ethically in alliance with their labels and marketing.

Well gosh, if it is "all-natural," it must be healthy, right? It actually may not be.

"Natural," "all-natural," or "100% natural" in the literal sense means no artificial ingredients or chemicals, indicating every single ingredient comes from Mother Nature.

What most people *don't* know is the term "natural" is not federally regulated. With the exception of the production of meat and poultry, there is no legal definition of "natural." The USDA definition of "natural" for meat and poultry defines it has no artificial or synthetic ingredients, including flavoring, coloring, or chemical preservative, and it must not be more than "minimally processed." This definition does not, however, govern the use of antibiotics, growth hormones, or pesticides. Animal welfare is also not indicated. This definition, however, does not extend beyond meat and poultry.

Found on their www.FDA.gov site, the FDA states,

> *"Although the FDA has not engaged in rulemaking to establish a formal definition for the term 'natural,' we do have a longstanding policy concerning the use of 'natural' in human food labeling. The FDA has considered the term 'natural' to mean that nothing artificial or synthetic (including all color additives regardless of source) has been included in, or has been added to, a food that would not normally be expected to be in that food. However, this policy was not intended to address food production methods, such as the use of pesticides, nor did it explicitly address food processing or manufacturing methods, such as thermal technologies, pasteurization, or irradiation. The FDA also did not consider whether the term 'natural' should describe any nutritional or other health benefit."*

Many well-known food companies have been cited for exploiting this very fact. They claim their products are "natural" when in fact those products contain synthetic preservatives like dimethicone or phenoxyethanol, pesticides, genetically modified organisms (GMOs), antibiotics, growth hormones, and artificial ingredients. Also, beware of products coming from other countries; they often have different standards regulating their ingredients and production practices.

In short, don't take the company's word for it. Be educated, and make the decision to buy based on *that* knowledge, not on the labeling and marketing.

RECAP

The term "natural" is not regulated and does not always mean natural... or healthy. Take a look at the ingredients list to see what is in there. The fewer ingredients, the simpler the product, the better.

38

"LOW FAT"

The words "low fat" or "light" are often eye-catching for people, especially those who are starting trying to eat well or lose weight. Imagine this: you're in the cookie aisle in the grocery store, and there are two varieties of the same cookie. The first variety is the regular you have had before, and the second looks very similar, except the packaging states the words "light" and "25% fewer calories." Well, that *must* be the better choice... right?

I'LL TAKE TWO PLEASE

In a study published in the Journal of Marketing Research, participants were given the choice of two bowls of M&M'S®: one was the "regular" version, and one was labelled "low fat." Interestingly, participants, on average, ate nearly 30% more of the "low fat" M&M'S®.

This type of marketing makes you *feel* like you are allowed to eat more of them to make up for the fewer calories per serving. It may actually serve you better to eat fewer of the full-fat M&M'S® than more of the low-fat M&M'S®.

This assumed nutritional benefit indicated by the "low fat" or "light" labeling should make you pause out of concern rather than drive your decision to buy.

REALITY CHECK

People succumb to the foods that *taste* good, and food companies are well aware of that fact. Fat equals flavor. If fat is being removed, what is being added to compensate?

The fewer calories or lower fat content—a.k.a. taking out the real ingredients that have the higher fat content—is often achieved by adding salt or sugar (usually synthetic and chemically man-made), artificial thickeners, and other unwanted, foreign ingredients to ensure the product still tastes "normal." What's ironic is these added ingredients that compensate for the reduction in fat and calories are usually more damaging to your health than the full-fat version.

Food for thought (pun intended): Why is fruit never labeled as "light?" Of course, that is a rhetorical question, but if the product you are wanting to buy that is labeled "light" is as healthy as they want you to think it is with their labeling, why should they need that label in the first place?

Usually if a product is high enough in fat or calories or otherwise seen as unhealthy, it probably has a slew of other qualities that *also* make it unhealthy, such as sugar, salt, or saturated fat content.

An additional thought on energy: What's the point of having something with less fat or fewer calories if it saps you of your energy while your body is trying to digest the crappy, man-made ingredients that are foreign to your body in the first place? You'll be more apt to not move as much (and therefore not burn as many calories) during the couple of hours immediately after eating it because of the extra energy and resources your body will need to just digest the artificial ingredients. Who wants to feel lethargic and unfocused?

WHAT TO DO

Instead of searching out the "low-fat" products, substitute the kind of product you were looking for with a similar product with better quality ingredients. The way to tell is to look at the ingredients list. If the ingredients list is a mile long with things you have either not heard of or stumble on when pronouncing them, it's probably not the most natural or wholesome food you could be fueling your body with. It will most likely bog you down from all the extra crap it is made with rather than give you energy.

RECAP

"Low fat" and "light" products usually have substitutes that do you more harm than good. And you will most likely eat more of the "low fat" products to unconsciously make up for the lower calorie content.

39

"DIET"

You may not control all the events that happen to you, but you can decide not to be reduced by them.
—MAYA ANGELOU

"Diet" anything usually refers to a reduction in the calorie content of a food or drink. So many different types of foods and drinks are also offered in a "diet" form, that it would be quite easy to live on mostly "diet" foods. Gosh, if you were calorie counting, you could have a field day! You could literally live on diet soda and baked potato chips and still be under 1000 calories each day. Why not, right? Since calorie-counting is now considered the "healthy" thing to do, you would be ultra-healthy!

I am being *extremely* sarcastic, and I hope you are picking up on that. If not, let me be very blunt. Do *not* rely on calorie counting as your gauge if an item is healthy. Do you know how miserable you would feel if that is all you consumed all day? Do you know how rough your body would run? How drained and disease-filled it would end up?

"Diet" anything usually means substitutions for the real ingredient *with* calories has taken place. This is usually achieved with manmade chemicals, fillers, and other ingredients foreign to your body. These manmade ingredients are chosen because they have no or very few calories in place of the legitimate, real foods that supply your body with calories (energy), nutrients, and vitamins.

DIET SODA = WEIGHT GAIN

Ah, the truth comes out.

Choosing diet soda is one of the first (and easiest) methods we think of to lose weight or get healthy. We proudly tout our cans of diet all over the place, proud with our choice, almost saying, "Look at me and my efforts to get healthy and lose weight." The eye-rolling can now commence.

If you are a diet soda drinker, I apologize for being so forward. If you truly love your diet soda and have it occasionally as more of a treat than a daily beverage and don't want to give it up, then please, continue on having it as an occasional treat. But I want to help. And I want to help by putting the thought that diet soda is a way to get healthy or a decent substitute for truly nutritious food or for physical activity, to a halt right here and now.

Diet soda does so many un-cool things to our bodies, it's not even close to funny. And it's amazing to me how many people are fooled by its perceived benefits.

Want to trick your body and make it all confused? Want to actually *gain* weight? Diet soda is a great way to do that. Allow me to explain...

People drink diet soda for the "benefit" of no calories and no sugar. But how does it still taste so sweet with no sugar? You probably already know that it is because of the chemical (artificial) sweeteners that are added in in place of the real caloric sugar.

What you may not know is this fake sugar tricks our taste buds by still satisfying a person's craving for the sweet taste and also tricks your body into thinking it's getting *real* food. Just *tasting* the fake sweetness releases insulin in your body, which drops your blood sugar, because it is expecting the real sugar spike. But it's just fake sugar. Without the actual sugar, your blood sugar stays low, which triggers more cravings for sugar because your body knows it needs to bring the blood sugar level back up.

Your body is an absolute pro at adapting to protect itself. Diet soda after diet soda, your body starts becoming used to not getting the type of food it's expecting and starts adapting the way it responds to protect itself from that drop in blood sugar.

Now the whole system is out of whack. When a diet soda drinker consumes *real* sugar, your body doesn't process it and react to it how it should because of how many times it has been tricked by the fake stuff... which means the body doesn't release the hormone that regulates the blood sugar. Now your blood sugar is all over the place, never knowing how it should react; your cravings are all over the place, trying to compensate for the all-over-the-place blood sugar levels; you start gaining weight, despite your "best efforts;" and you are confused and frustrated with the whole thing and give up on ever being healthy or losing weight or whatever your goal is. See how it snowballs? All from thinking "diet" was better.

CONCLUSION

*Identify your problems,
but give your power and energy to solutions.*
—TONY ROBBINS

It is easy for me to be eternally thankful for these mindful eating strategies and consistent exercise. Because of these, I have developed a standard of living for myself that kicked that teenage mentality of mine to the curb. I don't need to succumb to fad diets or have the guilt and shame I used to associate with overeating.

Binging, purging, dieting, and starving are no longer habits or fallbacks for me. If I do happen to eat too much, I feel bad, yes, but I also forgive myself and know my typical "90" part of my "90—10" lifestyle will even me back out.

I know myself well now. I know I go through stages of feeling "poufy." I am a woman; I get bloated during that certain time of month when I also happen to feel like crap and my hormonal perspective gets all out of whack. I also know I sometimes legitimately gain a few pounds when I have a few weeks of too many sweet cocktails or sugary coffees or fried foods and too little water.

How do I respond when this **season** happens, and what do I do?

Well, let me first say that I *do* feel like I have lost control during those times and feel frustrated with my body and the decisions.

And I *do* despise those feelings. Did you notice, though, that I called it a *season* of life?

Being aware of these feelings popping up is the first step. I don't want to go into reactive mode with emotion pushing the gas pedal. I slow it down, and I approach it logically.

I assure myself that I know the steps I need to take to right myself again, and my body knows what to do from there. I have to be aware in my frustrated mind to make sure my eating habits remain controlled and don't cross the line into a "diet" or over an even further line into "disordered." When I feel the bubbling of helplessness or hopelessness, that is when I remind myself it took weeks or months of too many cocktails, coffees, and pizza nights to gain the weight and pouf, and it will most likely take that long for my body to right itself with my more dialed in habits can't exercise the bloat away, and I certainly can't alcohol it away. I need to suck it up, own it, and **be patient**.

This being aware of your thoughts and feelings and being in control of both them and your eating habits is what I want for you, too. This is so much more in the realm of possibility than you think it is. Don't give up. Be patient. Love yourself and your body. Take it one eating habit at a time, and before long, you will have developed a standard of living that is indicative of a healthy lifestyle. Next step, exercise!

ACKNOWLEDGMENTS

There are special people in my life whose encouragement and assistance have made this book possible. I would like to send a very heartfelt acknowledgment to the following people for assisting me in the creation of this book:

Amy Tubbs
Andrea Schmalz
Angel Tollens
Becky Tollens—*thank you for the hours you spent typing suggestions!*
Brian Thompson
Charles Meyer
Claudine Mijal
Dawn Veley
Emerson Zentz
Jeff Thompson
Lindsay Thompson—*thank you Sister for your many hours writing your edits!*
Margaret Gabrick
Ross Gabrick
Sara Clark-Schroeder
Shawn Kincaid
Sherry Mijal—*thank you Mama for your hours of suggestions!*
Stan Holter
Stephanie Thompson
Tanya Leahy

FURTHER READING

Continue to follow Rachel's advice on not letting aspects of your health habits take over your life. The simple yet profound steps in her *Fitness for Life: The 6 Step System to Develop a Plan, Maintain Motivation, and Finally Make It Stick* book will forever change the way you approach and think about fitness:

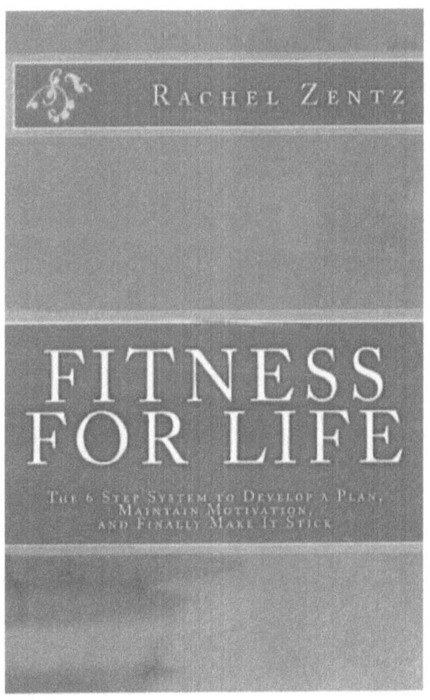

Type this in the address bar of your internet browser:
bit.ly/RachelZentzFitnessBook

FAVOR

Dear Reader,

THANK YOU FOR READING MY BOOK!

Can I ask a small favor of you?

IF you feel a little more in control of your eating…
IF you feel you are a little more able to enjoy your food…
IF you feel you are eating less…

Can I respectfully ask you to write a review for this book on Amazon? If you already have, thank you! If you haven't, I would really appreciate if you did so for me right now.

I value your feedback, and I love hearing what you have to say.

I need your input to make the next version of this book and my future books better. Here's how to do it:

1. Grab your phone.
2. Go to Amazon.com
3. Search "*Eat Less Enjoy More Rachel*"
4. Click on this book.
5. Click on "*Write a customer review*"

I look forward to reading it!

Sincerely and ever so gratefully,

Rachel

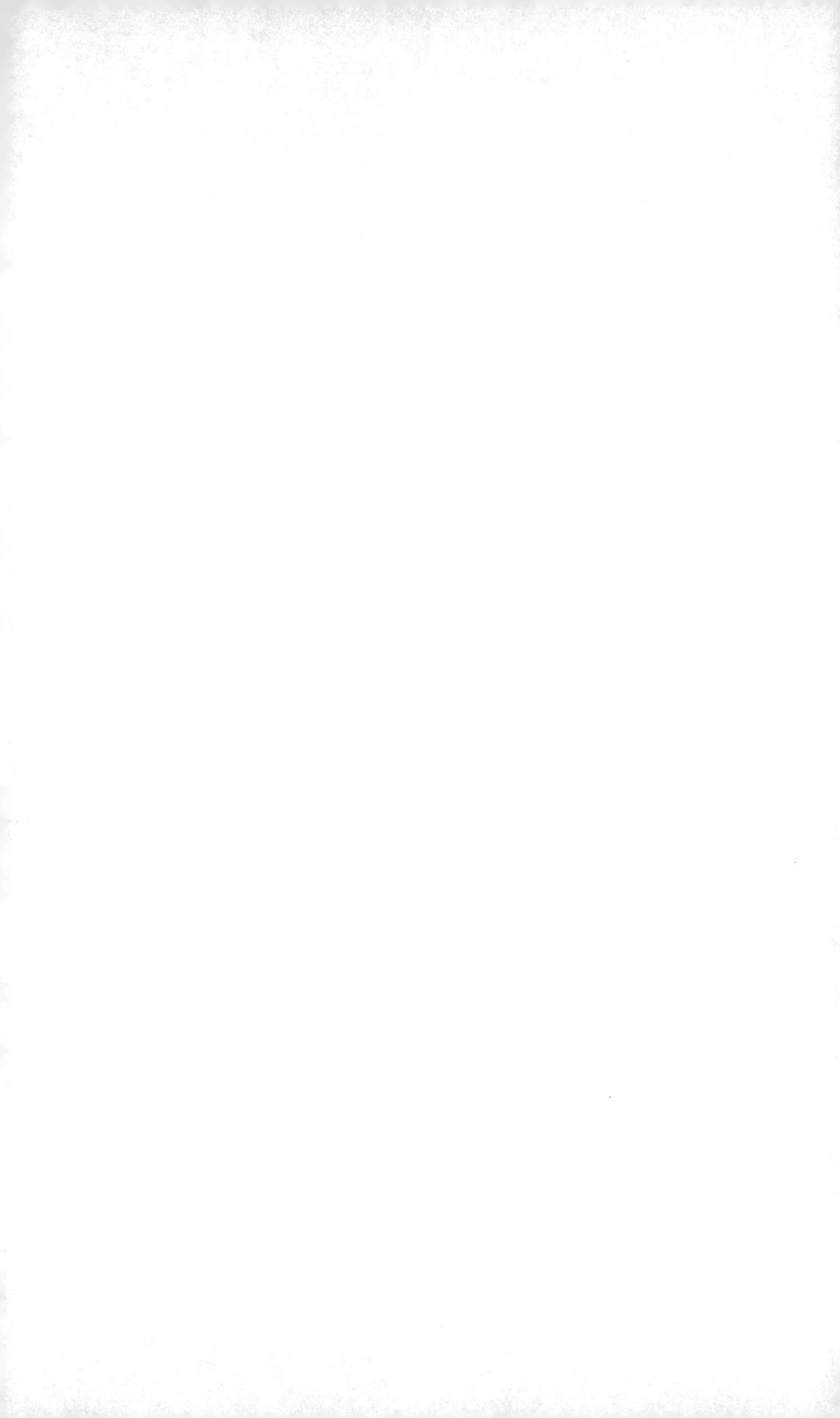

www.ingramcontent.com/pod-product-compliance
Lightning Source LLC
Chambersburg PA
CBHW031228250726
48655CB00005B/1852